COLORADO CLEANSE

14 Day Ayurvedic Detox and Digestive Rejuvenation

Also by John Douillard

Books

Body, Mind and Sport
The Mind-Body Guide to Lifelong Health, Fitness, and Your Personal Best

Perfect Health for Kids
10 Ayurvedic Health Secrets Every Parent Must Know

The 3-Season Diet
Eat the Way Nature Intended: Lose Weight, Beat Food Cravings, Get Fit

The Encyclopedia of Ayurvedic Massage

The Yoga Body Diet
Slim and Sexy in 4 Weeks Without the Stress

DVDs

Ayurveda for Detox

Ayurveda for Stress Relief

Ayurveda for Weight Loss

eCourses

28-Day Ayurveda Challenge
Change Your Daily Routine, Change Your Life

John Douillard's Ayurvedic Pulse Reading Course
A Technique for Self-Discovery

Available at LifeSpa.com

COLORADO CLEANSE

14 Day Ayurvedic Detox and Digestive Rejuvenation

John Douillard

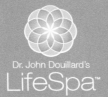

Dr. John Douillard's
LifeSpa™

This book may be purchased for business or promotional use for special sales. For information, please contact us.

Internet addresses given in this book were accurate at the time of publication.

Published by LifeSpa Products™, LLC in the United States of America

First Edition – May 2010

Second Edition – August 2011

Third Edition – August 2013

Cover and Book Design by Vladimir Mirkovic

ISBN: 978-0-9898242-9-3

John Douillard's LifeSpa

6662 Gunpark Drive E, Suite 102
Boulder, CO 80301
(303) 516 – 4848
lifespa.com | info@lifespa.com

To Ginger
The love of my life!

Contents

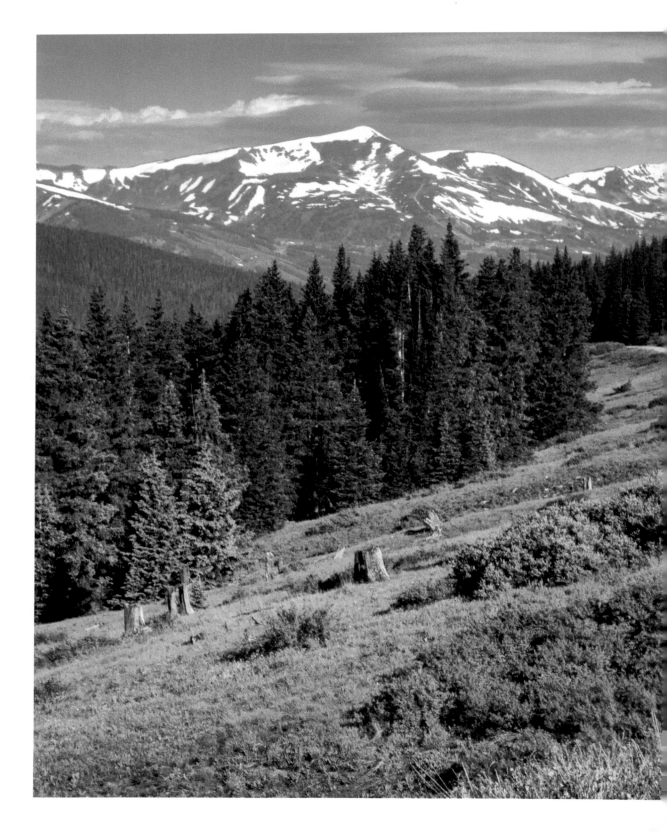

Introduction

What You'll Need
Day-by-Day Guide

Congratulations. You are about to embark on a life-changing journey towards health and vibrancy. A few years ago, after almost 30 years of guiding folks through Ayurvedic detoxes and retreats, I developed a home detox called the Colorado Cleanse. The results have been nothing short of remarkable.

In my early twenties, fascinated by longevity experts, I started doing fasting and colon cleanses to be vital at 100. While I always felt great after each cleanse, I soon became dependent on cleansing, needing to cleanse regularly to feel and digest well. After years of cleansing and ultimately studying Ayurveda, it became clear that you cannot detox well if you cannot digest well. So I started my quest to rebuild my broken digestive system. Today, while I have better digestion at 57 than I've ever had before, I still feel my digestion getting better with each Colorado Cleanse I do.

Why cleanse?

You're probably already aware that we live in a toxic world at the moment. Most of America is covered by coal mine plumes that drop mercury on all our organic veggies. On top of that, there are preservatives, pesticides, plastics, and environmental pollutants that we cannot avoid.

While we have the ability to detoxify most of these chemicals, it simply does not happen unless you have a good strong digestive system. For example, to digest gluten, dairy and fried foods well, you need a strong digestive system. Avoiding these foods altogether may be a healthier choice, but it may also mean that your digestive/detox strength is compromised and you are at greater risk of toxicity. Basically, if you can't digest gluten or a high-fat meal, how are you going to digest and then detox the mercury on your organic spinach?

The Colorado Cleanse resets digestive strength before beginning the detox process, because the detoxification pathways are the same in the body as the digestive pathways. Many folks who could not eat wheat and dairy due to weak digestion can now digest these hard to digest foods. Perhaps more importantly, they have optimized their natural ability to detoxify the body in spite of our toxic world.

What are toxins?

Some of the pollutant molecules we are exposed to are fat-soluble, while others are water-soluble. Our bodies are pretty good at detoxing water-soluble toxins. The kidneys typically flush them out with our liquid waste.

Fat-soluble toxins are trickier and require multiple phases of detoxification by the liver. Often the liver is already overwhelmed and diverts these fat-soluble toxins into the blood. Since they are lipophilic – meaning attracted to other fats – they pick fat cells around your belly, hips or even your brain to bind to and store in – in some cases for decades.

All cleanses hope to pull toxins out of the fat cells. The question is: where do the toxins go from there? The body stores toxins in the fat when it cannot digest and process them properly. If you do not reset your digestive strength before you cleanse, you risk just moving the toxins from one fat cell to another and feeling worse.

The 3 phases of the Colorado Cleanse.

The Colorado Cleanse is a unique detox and digestive reset program that operates in three phases.

Phase 1 is a 4-day Pre-Cleanse in which we will prime the digestive tract by scrubbing it out with supportive herbs and a high-fiber, low-fat diet. This will also thin the bile, which will help decongest the liver and pancreatic ducts, which become congested over time. We'll also be opening up the detox channels and getting them cleared and ready to move toxins in Phase 2. Think of this phase as pushing back the curtains, opening the windows wide, and getting ready to do some deep cleaning.

Phase 2 is the Main Cleanse, which lasts 7 days. This is when we get into fat metabolism – the mechanism by which we will coax toxins out of the fat cells and into the colon for elimination. During this phase, we again boost liver and gallbladder function and continue to reset all aspects of digestion and elimination. The main cleanse will support healthy lymphatic flow, balanced blood sugar and reset your ability to burn fat-soluble toxins long after the cleanse is over.

In Phase 3, once the digestive tract is cleaned out and reset, we'll focus on stoking and resetting the digestive fire. This phase is also your antidote to the binge-after-fasting phenomenon. It's so easy to come off a cleanse only to indulge in hard-to-digest toxic foods again, which can make you feel worse than when you started. Phase 3 is a Post-Cleanse designed to make sure that your re-entry into non-cleanse eating isn't a shock to you or your digestion.

This is not a starvation cleanse.

After years of trying out different cleanses, I've come to realize that you don't have to starve to give your body a good detox. In fact, starving is one of the surest ways to send the body into emergency mode. In this mode, the body clings to fat as a survival fuel, clinging to the toxins right along with it.

The truth is, **the body has to feel safe** to effectively burn fat and detoxify. So much of how we implement the Colorado Cleanse is based on that principle. Through a methodical though still nourishing diet and some proven lifestyle techniques that anyone can do, we will disarm the central nervous system by convincing it that the stress war is over and it's safe to burn fat and release old toxins.

In addition to being nourished the entire time and having permission to eat as much as you need to stay full, you will have three different Meal Options during Phase 2 of this cleanse – ranging from the option that includes the widest array of foods to the most austere option – which is a mono-diet of the traditional Ayurvedic healing food kitchari, an ultra-digestible blend of basmati rice and split yellow mung dahl beans cooked to a soft, soupy consistency. In the vein of not stressing, I recommend starting with the most diverse Meal Option (3 – "Nourish") first and moving towards the most austere (1 – "Transform") as you become more comfortable. If this means that you stay on the most diverse option for the entire cleanse, that is absolutely fine and you will still get all the benefits.

You will become a better cleanser every time.

Chances are you will do this cleanse more than once. In fact, most people that do it once go on to do it biannually during the transitional seasons of spring and fall, as is traditional to Ayurveda. This isn't any persuasive genius on my part – the truth is that most of us feel refreshed on every level after doing this cleanse, and notice significant improvements that build with each subsequent cleanse. Most of us begin to crave these results naturally.

Emotional release.

Research at the National Institutes of Health (NIH) has found that our emotions, in the traceable and measurable form of what is now referred to as "molecules of emotion," are carried by peptides all over the body. Old toxic negative emotions were found to block the flow of the body's information network and cause disease, according to the NIH.[1]

Thousands of years ago, Ayurveda created cleansing procedures to detoxify toxic emotions that store in the fat and muscle of the body. The Colorado Cleanse incorporates this emotional layer of toxic buildup into its detox plan. It is designed to release these molecules of emotion from the fat cells and give us the opportunity for deep transformational change through a series of specific Self-Inquiry exercises that you'll be working with in Phase 2.

Your Microbiology

The body is made up of trillions of cells, but only 10% of them are human. The other 90% are microbial cells, and the vast majority of them live in the digestive tract. They are responsible for immunity, detox, mood, evolutionary changes to DNA and just about every other human function. They are the 90%!

To optimize your health, we must create the perfect environment for the good microbes to thrive. The Colorado Cleanse does its part in this by resetting digestive function – which is critical for the

---

1   Pert, C. *Molecules of Emotion*. 1997 Simon and Schuster.

proliferation of diverse strains of good bugs.

Don't strain – this is not an endurance event.

As I mentioned above, our bodies only know how to do one thing well when we are stressed – hold on to fat. During this cleanse, I am challenging you to let go. Let go of the need to do it perfectly, of the desire to do the most austere Meal Option right away or to do all of the Optional Stress-Relief Practices if you don't have time (self-care practices can easily turn to self-berating practices if we are pushing ourselves too hard). You get the picture.

Here is your mantra for the Colorado Cleanse:

> Relax. Do the best you can. The rest will come.

Be Non-GMO and Organic on this cleanse and beyond.

One of the biggest new threats to our health are genetically modified foods – or GMO's. These foods have been shown to be of inferior nutritional content to their non-GMO counterparts, as well as to wreak havoc on the precious micro-ecology of beneficial bacteria in the digestive tract.

Since this is not a starvation cleanse, it's critical that all the foods that we do consume in the next two weeks are organic – meaning they aren't treated with synthetic pesticides or fertilizers – and non-GMO. Some foods are more likely to be genetically engineered than others. In Appendix 1 of this book, you will find a list of Foods to Avoid that highlights which foods to be most aware of when looking for non-GMO.

Please consider taking the time to educate yourself on this issue, and committing to a non-GMO diet for the duration of this cleanse and for the rest of your life.

I hope you enjoy this cleanse as much as I do each time I do it.

Bye for now,
John Douillard

What You'll Need

As with any cleanse, you will need some supplies. Here, I've broken up the supply list into what you'll need for each phase, followed by a short list of supplies you'll need across all the phases. If you find yourself overwhelmed by the amount of supplies, just remember that your grocery bill for the next two weeks will be much smaller than usual.

The following lists are based on the amounts for 1 person. Multiply as needed for any fellow cleansers in your household.

Phase 1 (Pre-Cleanse)

Apples

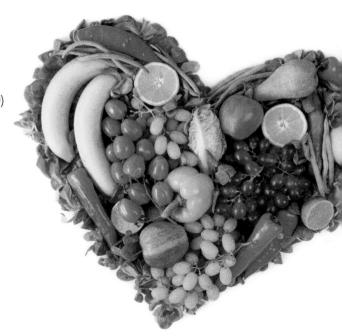

- 12 – 20 organic, non-GMO apples
  (For unstable blood sugar replace
  with Malic Acid, see bottom of page 60)

Beet Tonic Ingredients

- 4 – 8 fresh beets
- 4 lemons
- Dijon mustard (optional)

Green Tonic Ingredients

- 6 stalks celery
- 2 cups fresh parsley
- 4 cups string beans
- 4 zucchini

Meals

- Grains, legumes, seeds, fruits and vegetables for your meals. Peruse the recipes in Chapter 17 and buy ingredients for those that appeal to you.

Optional

- Organic rice cakes
- 2 – 4 avocados

Phase 2 (Main Cleanse)

Ghee

- Regular dosages: 8 oz. of ghee
- Advanced dosages: 16 oz. of ghee
- Optional: Rice, almond, coconut, or organic vat-pasteurized, non-homogenized cow's milk to take with the ghee during Phase 2. (If using coconut, look for the milk-alternative kind normally sold in a carton – NOT the fatty coconut "cream" sold in cans).

Kitchari
For Transform, Rejuvenate, and Nourish Meal Options (see chapter 12 to find your Meal Option)

- Approximately 10 packets of LifeSpa's Organic Kitchari
  OR
- 4 lbs of split yellow mung dahl beans, 4 lbs of basmati rice, and spices (suggested cleansing spices: organic coriander seed, organic cumin seed, organic black mustard seed, organic turmeric, organic fennel seed, sea salt).

For Rejuvenate Meal Option, add:

- Seasonal vegetables for steaming*

For Nourish Meal Option, add:

- Seasonal vegetables for steaming*
- Seasonal greens and veggies for eating as a salad* (in the spring/summer)
- Gluten-free oats
- Seasonal Fruits*

If adding protein

- Lean chicken or turkey and/or a low-fat protein powder of your choice (concentrates are better than isolates).

Final Flush
- 1 – 1.5 Tablespoon Epsom salts, 1 lemon, and 2 Tablespoon olive oil
  OR
- 1 ½ cups prune juice (for sensitive digestion)

Phase 3 (Post-Cleanse)

- **Grains, legumes, seeds, fruits and veggies for your meals.** Peruse the recipes in Chapter 17 and buy ingredients for those that appeal to you.
- 12 lemons
- Note: If you liked the Beet Tonic and Green Tonic, you may certainly continue them during Phase 3, but they are not required.

For All Phases

Herbs**

- Digestive Formula: Warm or Cool Digest
- Sugar Destroyer
- Beet Cleanse
- Manjistha
- Turmeric Plus
- Liver Repair
- Regenerate

> **Colorado Cleanse Kit**
>
> Colorado Cleanse supply kits are available in the online store at LifeSpa.com/ColoradoCleanse

Abhyanga Self-Massage

- LifeSpa's Lymphatic Massage Oil or sesame oil (see page 55 for instructions on curing sesame oil).

---

* See Appendix 2 of this book for a list of Seasonal Cleansing Foods.

**See Chapter 5 for alternatives to these herbal formulas.

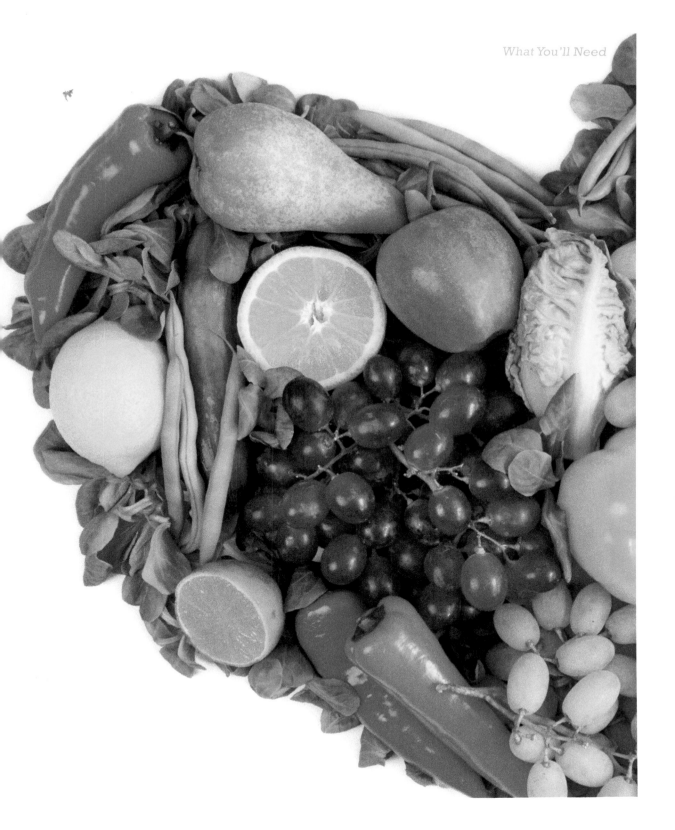

2 Day-by-Day Guide

Phase 1

Phase 1: Day 1

Preparation
Please see the Shopping List for Phase 1 in the "What You'll Need" chapter (page 14).

What to Eat

- Each day eat: 1-2 Beet Tonics, 1-2 Green Tonics, and 3-5 apples eaten after meals.
- Eat a low-fat, whole, unprocessed food, seasonal diet of whole grains, legumes, soup, salad, fruit, vegetables and seeds (recipes on page 92). Add lean meat or a soy-free protein drink if needed (see details on adding protein on page 37).
- See the Foods to Avoid list in Appendix 1.
- Eat 3 meals a day without snacking. If you are used to grazing, start with 4 meals per day and work towards 3. Eat enough at each meal to carry you through to the next meal.

Before Meal Herbs	After Meal Herbs
Take 1 capsule of each 15 minutes *before* each meal, 3 times per day, with 12 oz. of warm water.	**Take 1 capsule of each** 15 minutes *after* each meal, 3 times per day, with 12 oz. of warm water.
• Sugar Destroyer	• Manjistha
• Beet Cleanse	• Turmeric Plus
• Warm or Cool Digest	• Regenerate
	• Liver Repair

See Chapter 5 on page 40 for more details about the herbs and their alternatives.

Sample Menu for Day 1

- Breakfast: creamed millet cereal, cinnamon and hemp seeds followed by 1 -2 apples.

- Lunch: Black Bean and Quinoa Burrito (wrapped in greens) with guacamole and Beet Tonic. 1 -2 apples after the meal.

- Dinner: Savory Green Tonic Soup with Red Rice (beets and rice), Beet Tonic and 1 rice cake with avocado. 1 apple after the meal.

- With each meal, sip hot water or a non-caffeinated herbal tea.

Rehydration Therapy

- Hot Sips: Do your best to sip plain hot water throughout the day
(2-3 sips every 10-15 minutes).
- Daily Ounces: Do your best to drink ½ your ideal body weight in ounces of plain water.

12-Minute Workout
(see chapter 6 for a detailed description)

Optional Stress-Relief Practices
(see chapter 7 for detailed descriptions of each of the following practices)

- Yoga, 2-3 times today (15 minutes each)
- Breathing, 2-3 times today (10 minutes each)
- Meditation, 2-3 times today (10 minutes each)
- Daily Self-Massage (5 minutes)

Having Trouble?

- Stop or reduce the dose of the herbs. Once you are feeling better, restart the herbs at 1 capsule each day with the main meal (lunch), then slowly work up to 1 capsule with each meal if comfortable.
- Drink more water.
- Eat more protein: lean meat or soy-free protein drink.

Phase 1: Day 2

Follow all the instructions for Day 1 on page 18.

Sample Menu for Day 2

- Breakfast: Green Tonic with sunflower seeds followed by 1-2 apples.

- Lunch: Tuscan Soup (white beans with kale) and Rosemary-Garlic Rice and Beet Tonic. 1-2 apples after the meal.

- Dinner: One Pot Lentils and Rice with Beet-Ginger Salad. 1 apple after the meal.

- With each meal, sip hot water or a non-caffeinated herbal tea.

Phase 1: Day 3

Follow all the instructions for Day 1 on page 18.

Sample Menu for Day 3

- Breakfast: Green Tonic with pumpkin seeds followed by 1-2 apples.

- Lunch: Colorful Lunch (avocado-tomato salad with beet soup, seeds, and steamed veggies) and Beet Tonic. 1-2 apples after the meal.

- Dinner: Savory Green Tonic Soup with rice cake and avocado. 1 apple after the meal.

- With each meal, sip hot water or a non-caffeinated herbal tea.

Phase 1: Day 4

Follow all the instructions for Day 1 on page 18.

Sample Menu for Day 4

- Breakfast: Steel cut oatmeal* cooked with ginger, cardamom and garnished with pumpkin seeds. 1-2 apples after the meal.

- Lunch: Moroccan Lentil Stew with Beet Greens and Moroccan Beet Salad. 1-2 apples after the meal.

- Dinner: Mexican Squash Mash with guacamole, Spanish Quinoa and Beet Tonic. 1 apple after the meal.

- With each meal, sip hot water or a non-caffeinated herbal tea.

Buy steel cut oats that are Certified Gluten-Free or "not contaminated with wheat".

Phase 2

Phase 2: Day 5

Preparation
Please see the Shopping List for Phase 2 in the "What You'll Need" chapter (page 15).

What to Eat

- Eat a nonfat diet. Avoid all fats: nuts, seeds, avocado, oil, dairy, fried foods, etc.
- Start with Nourish (Meal Option #3), which includes kitchari, whole grains, legumes, steamed veggies, salad and lean protein. Eat seasonally.
- Move to the Rejuvenate and/or Transform Meal Options only when your blood sugar is stable. See the Meal Options on page 72 and recipes on page 92.
- See the Foods to Avoid list in Appendix 1.
- Eat 3 meals a day without snacking. If you are used to grazing, start with 4 meals per day and work towards 3. Eat enough at each meal to carry you through to the next meal.

Morning Ghee

Please note: Only ingest the amount of ghee that is easy for you to digest and is comfortable. If you have gallbladder trouble or difficulty digesting fats, drink only 2-3 teaspoons (or less) of ghee every morning and do not increase ghee dosages.

1. First thing each morning when you wake up, drink the suggested amount of melted ghee. It is best to do this as early in the morning as possible on an empty stomach.
2. Slowly melt the teaspoons of ghee in a pot over low heat.
3. Drink on an empty stomach.
4. Wait ½ hour before drinking or eating anything so that the ghee has time to collect toxins.
5. You do not need to take the Warm Digest or Cool Digest before the ghee – take it only before your meals. If you feel full after the ghee and do not need breakfast, you can skip the morning dose of herbs as well.

Ghee Dosages for Day 5

- Regular: 2 tsp. of ghee

- Advanced: 3 tsp. of ghee

Special Tips for the Morning Ghee

- If it's difficult for you to drink plain melted ghee, add a ½ cup of warm rice, almond, coconut, or organic vat-pasteurized, non-homogenized cow's milk. Warm the ghee and the "milk" to the same temperature so they mix easily and then drink it all at once. If needed, you can add a pinch of nutmeg, cinnamon and/or cardamom.
- Try holding your nose while sipping the ghee.
- Use flax seed, coconut or olive oil if you cannot use ghee (read chapter 11 for more on ghee and viable alternatives).
- If nausea occurs, sip ½ - 1 cup of warm-to-hot water with fresh lemon juice and grated ginger root. Eat a little kitchari ½ hour after drinking the ghee even if you feel full. This helps settle the stomach. Take less ghee the next morning.
- Only increase the dose of ghee each day if you are tolerating it. If you experience loose, uncomfortable stools then do not increase the dose of ghee the next morning. Decrease the ghee to a dose that is comfortable for you. Stay at the current dose until you are comfortable and then increase. Remember - Do Not Strain.

Before Meal Herbs	After Meal Herbs
Take 1 capsule of each 15 minutes *before* each meal, 3 times per day, with 12 oz. of warm water.	**Take 1 capsule of each** 15 minutes *after* each meal, 3 times per day, with 12 oz. of warm water.
• Sugar Destroyer	• Manjistha
• Beet Cleanse	• Turmeric Plus
• Warm or Cool Digest	• Regenerate
	• Liver Repair

See Chapter 5 for more details about the herbs and their alternatives.

Rehydration Therapy

- Hot Sips: Do your best to sip plain hot water throughout the day
  (2-3 sips every 10-15 minutes).
- Daily Ounces: Do your best to drink ½ your ideal body weight in ounces of plain water.

12-Minute Workout (see chapter 6 for a detailed description)

Self-Inquiry

- See page 78 for instructions on today's Self-Inquiry exercises.

Optional Stress-Relief Practices
(see chapter 7 for detailed descriptions of each of the following practices)

- Yoga, 2-3 times today (15 minutes each)
- Breathing, 2-3 times today (10 minutes each)
- Meditation, 2-3 times today (10 minutes each)
- Daily Self-Massage (5 minutes)

Having Trouble?

- Stop or reduce the dose of the herbs. Once you are feeling better, restart the herbs at 1
  capsule each day with lunch, then slowly work up to 1 capsule with each meal if comfortable.
- Drink more water.
- Take less ghee, or stop the ghee.
  If you stop the ghee, add seeds or avocado to your meal option.
- Follow the Nourish meal option and eat more protein,
  such as lean meat or soy-free protein drink.

Phase 2: Day 6

Follow all the instructions for Day 5 on page 22.

Ghee Dosages for Day 6

- Regular: 4 tsp. of ghee

- Advanced: 6 tsp. of ghee

Self-Inquiry - See page 78 for instructions on today's Self-Inquiry exercises.

Phase 2: Day 7

Follow all the instructions for Day 5 on page 22.

Ghee Dosages for Day 7

- Regular: 4 tsp. of ghee

- Advanced: 9 tsp. of ghee

Self-Inquiry - See page 78 for instructions on today's Self-Inquiry exercises.

Phase 2: Day 8

Follow all the instructions for Day 5 on page 22.

Ghee Dosages for Day 8

- Regular: 6 tsp. of ghee

- Advanced: 12 tsp. of ghee

Self-Inquiry - See page 78 for instructions on today's Self-Inquiry exercises.

Phase 2: Day 9

Follow all the instructions for Day 5 on page 22.

Ghee Dosages for Day 9

- Regular: 8 tsp. of ghee

- Advanced: 15 tsp. of ghee

Self-Inquiry - See page 78 for instructions on today's Self-Inquiry exercises.

Phase 2: Day 10

Follow all the instructions for Day 5 on page 22.

Ghee Dosages for Day 10

- Regular: 8 tsp. of ghee

- Advanced: 18 tsp. of ghee

Self-Inquiry - See page 78 for instructions on today's Self-Inquiry exercises.

Phase 2: Day 11

Follow all the instructions for Day 5 on page 22.

Ghee Dosages for Day 11

- Regular: 10 tsp. of ghee

- Advanced: 21 tsp. of ghee

Self-Inquiry - See page 78 for instructions on today's Self-Inquiry exercises.

Final Flush on the Evening of Day 11 (see chapter 14 for a detailed description)

Phase 3

Phase 3: Day 12

Preparation
Please see the Shopping List for Phase 3 on page 16 of the "What You'll Need" chapter.

What to Eat

- Eat a low-fat, whole food, seasonal diet of whole grains, legumes, soup, salad, vegetables and seeds (recipes on page 92). Add lean meat or a soy-free protein drink if needed.
- Optional: continue eating the Beet Tonic, Green Tonic, and apples - only if you enjoy them.
- See the Foods to Avoid list in Appendix 1.
- Eat 3 meals a day without snacking. If you are used to grazing, start with 4 meals per day and work towards 3. Eat enough at each meal to carry you through to the next meal.

Before Meal Herbs	After Meal Herbs
Take each before meal herb 15 minutes *before* each meal, 3 times per day, with 12 oz. of lemon water. Sip 4 more ounces of lemon water during the meal. (To make the lemon water, mix the juice of 1 lemon in 16 oz. of water.)	**Take 1 capsule of each after meal herb** 15 minutes *after* each meal, 3 times per day, with 12 oz. of warm water.
• 1 capsule Sugar Destroyer	• Manjistha
• NEW: 2 capsules Beet Cleanse	• Turmeric Plus
• NEW: 2 capsules Warm or Cool Digest	• Regenerate
	• Liver Repair

See Chapter 5 for more details about the herbs and their alternatives.

Rehydration Therapy

- Hot Sips: Do your best to sip plain hot water throughout the day (2-3 sips every 10-15 minutes).
- Daily Ounces: Do your best to drink ½ your ideal body weight in ounces of plain water.

12-Minute Workout
(see chapter 6 for a detailed description)

Optional Stress-Relief Practices
(see chapter 7 for detailed descriptions of each of the following practices)

- Yoga, 2-3 times today (15 minutes each)
- Breathing, 2-3 times today (10 minutes each)
- Meditation, 2-3 times today (10 minutes each)
- Daily Self-Massage (5 minutes)

Having Trouble?

- Stop or reduce the dose of the herbs. Once you are feeling better, restart the herbs at 1 capsule each day with lunch, and then slowly work up to 1 capsule with each meal if comfortable.
- Drink more water.
- Eat more protein: lean meat or soy-free protein drink.

Phase 3: Day 13

Follow all the instructions for Day 12 on page 27.

Before Meal Herbs	After Meal Herbs
Take each before meal herb	**Take 1 capsule of each after meal herb**
15 minutes *before* each meal, 3 times per day, with 12 oz. of lemon water. Sip 4 more ounces of lemon water during the meal. (To make the lemon water, mix the juice of 1 lemon in 16 oz. of water.)	15 minutes *after* each meal, 3 times per day, with 12 oz. of warm water.
	• Manjistha
• 1 capsule Sugar Destroyer	• Turmeric Plus
• NEW: 3 capsules Beet Cleanse	• Regenerate
• NEW: 3 capsules Warm or Cool Digest	• Liver Repair

See Chapter 5 for more details about the herbs and their alternatives.

Phase 3: Day 14

Follow all the instructions for Day 12 on page 27.

Before Meal Herbs	After Meal Herbs
Take each before meal herb 15 minutes *before* each meal, 3 times per day, with 12 oz. of lemon water. Sip 4 more ounces of lemon water during the meal. (To make the lemon water, mix the juice of 1 lemon in 16 oz. of water.)	**Take 1 capsule of each after meal herb** 15 minutes *after* each meal, 3 times per day, with 12 oz. of warm water.
• 1 capsule Sugar Destroyer	• Manjistha
• NEW: 4 capsules Beet Cleanse	• Turmeric Plus
• NEW: 4 capsules Warm or Cool Digest	• Regenerate
	• Liver Repair

See Chapter 5 for more details about the herbs.

Integration - After the Colorado Cleanse

For the next month, and as best as you can in the future, eat a normal diet with an emphasis on seasonally harvested foods. See chapter 16 for more about Integration and eating seasonally.

If you wish to continue the benefits you have received, eat a whole food, sugar- and sweetener-free diet without processed foods or cooked oils for as long as it is comfortable.

To further rebuild the digestive villi and colonize new, healthy diverse strains of intestinal microbes in the gut, consider taking:

- 2 packets each day of Gut Revival for 1 month.
- Followed by 1 capsule each day of Flora Restore for 2 months.
- Or take a probiotic that has been proven to endure digestive acids and adhere to the gut wall and includes these strains: *Bifidobacterium lactis, Lactobacillus acidophilus, Lactobacillus plantarum,* and *Bifidobacterium longum.*

Before Meal Herbs – Finish the Bottles	After Meal Herbs – Finish the Bottles
Take 1 capsule of each (or alternative) 15 minutes before each meal, 3 times per day, with 12 oz. of warm water.	**Take 1 capsule of each (or alternative)** 15 minutes *after* each meal, 3 times per day, with 12 oz. of warm water.
• Sugar Destroyer	• Manjistha
• Beet Cleanse	• Turmeric Plus
• Warm or Cool Digest	• Regenerate
	• Liver Repair

See Chapter 5 for more details about the herbs.

Take Warm or Cool Digest as needed, before a late or heavy meal.

12-Minute Workout (see chapter 6 for a detailed description)

Optional Stress-Relief Practices
(see chapter 7 for detailed descriptions of each of the following practices)

- Yoga, once per day if possible (15 minutes)
- Breathing, once per day if possible (10 minutes)
- Meditation, once per day if possible (10 minutes)
- Daily Self-Massage is optional (5 minutes)

Learn more:
For more information about transitioning to 3 meals a day without snacks, eating with the seasons, and recipe ideas, read my books:

The 3-Season Diet (lifespa.com/3seasondiet)

The Yoga Body Diet (lifespa.com/yogabody)

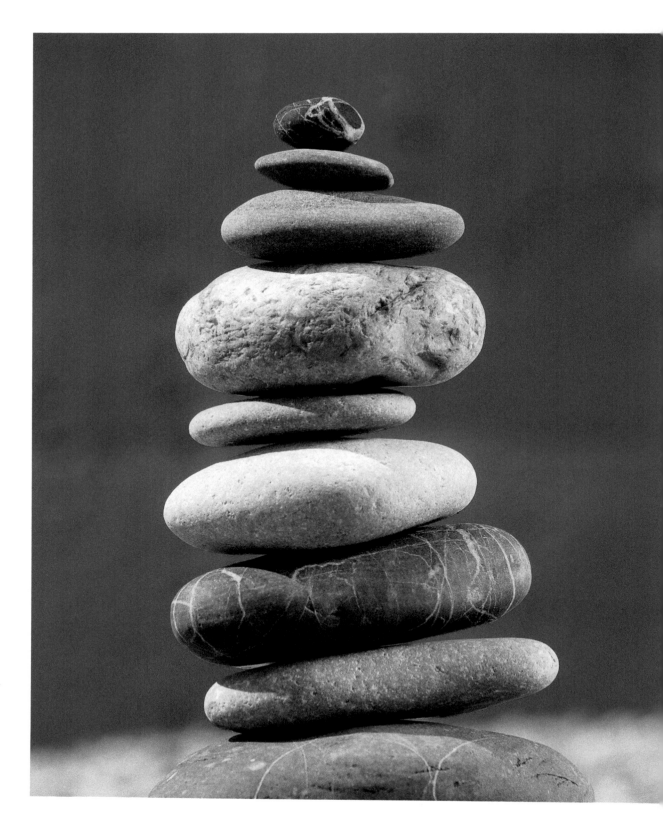

Essential Guidelines

3 Meals a Day
Rehydration
Herbs
12-Minute Workout
Optional Stress-Relief Practices

3) 3 Meals a Day

During the Colorado Cleanse, we are asking you to do something that you just might fall in love with and do for the rest of your life: **eat 3 meals a day with no snacks in between.**

Many of us have trained our bodies to rely on snacks or small meals every few hours or less. This tells the body that there is a constant supply of energy coming in, and that there is no reason to burn its stored fat.

Burning stored fat is important even if you aren't trying to lose weight. Our fat cells are where toxins are stored, so as long as we are ingesting enough good fats in our regular lives and eating an adequate balanced diet, burning fat between meals will not result in excessive weight loss, although it is an incredibly effective way to find and maintain a healthy, balanced weight.

Why You Want to Become a Fantastic Fat Burner

Fat is a calm, stable, non-emergency fuel. When you are in fat burning mode, your body gets the message that the stress war is over, and begins to relax. This benefit is difficult to overemphasize in a culture that is plagued by stress.

Fat burning also:

- Neutralizes acidity in the body

- Detoxifies fat-soluble toxins that can store in our fat cells for 20 years of more!

- Detoxifies fat-soluble molecules of emotion that lock us into repetitive detrimental patterns of thinking, feeling and behaving

- Stimulates lymphatic drainage

- Helps naturally maintain a healthy weight

How to Transition to 3 Meals a Day

If you are used to snacking or have adopted a diet of frequent small meals, eating 3 meals a day will require a transition. Here are some tips to ease in:

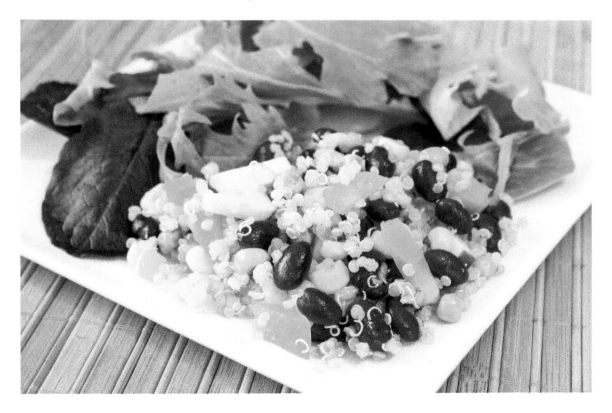

- Start with 4 meals with no snacks in between and gradually work towards 3 meals a day.
- Make each meal psychologically satisfying by stopping, sitting down, and enjoying each bite.
- Eat enough food at breakfast to carry you through to lunch.
- Eat a big, warm, satisfying lunch between the hours of 10am and 2pm. In Ayurveda, it is believed that lunch should be the biggest meal of the day. Eat enough to carry you through to supper.
- Eat a light, early supper – think of supper as "supplemental" to your midday meal, rather than a big standalone meal. That said, do eat enough supper to carry you through the night until breakfast without hunger (if you are not sleeping well, it may mean you need to eat more at supper).

Blood Sugar Balancing

Blood sugar crashes are not uncommon in the first days of the cleanse, especially if you are shooting for 3 meals a day with no snacks after having lived a lifestyle that relies heavily on snacks and/or small, frequent meals.

It can even happen in Phase 2 of the cleanse, and sometimes quite suddenly, even after having done well for a few days before. Stress, not-quite-right timing of meals, or not eating enough at your previous meal can all be insidious reasons for a blood sugar crash.

Keep a watchful eye out for the following symptoms, which can onset abruptly:

- Headaches
- Shakiness
- Nervousness or anxiety
- Sweating, chills and clamminess
- Irritability or impatience
- Confusion, including delirium
- Rapid/fast heartbeat
- Lightheadedness or dizziness
- Hunger and nausea
- Sleepiness
- Blurred/impaired vision
- Tingling or numbness in the lips or tongue
- Weakness or fatigue
- Anger, stubbornness, or sadness
- Lack of coordination
- Nightmares or crying out during sleep
- Seizures
- Unconsciousness

As you can see, keeping your blood sugar balanced is vital. The important thing is to know what to do when it happens – and not to panic. This does not mean you failed at the cleanse, or that the cleanse is over.

The first thing to do is to have a snack.

That's right, scrap the rules this one time and have a nonfat healthy snack. During Phase 2, the best option is a small bowl of kitchari. The next best option, and a viable option in any of the phases, is an apple, as it will still deliver some of the benefits we are looking for from this cleanse. If you don't have an apple on hand, another fruit or a vegetable is the next best option.

The second thing to do is to add protein to your future meals.

If in Phase 2, replace the rice in your kitchari with quinoa or, if you are using pre-mixed packets of kitchari, you can add a ½ cup of quinoa to the contents of one packet of kitchari. Quinoa has more protein than rice and will give your kitchari a protein kick.

If you eat meat, add some lean chicken to your next meal and each midday meal thereafter (or each meal, if you need) until you feel your blood sugar stabilize.

If you don't eat meat, add a small (8 oz.) protein shake to your next meal and with each midday meal thereafter (or each meal, if you need) until you feel your blood sugar stabilize. It can be whey, pea, hemp, or rice protein, but try for a concentrate rather than an isolate (look for this in the Nutrition Facts on the label).

If you are in Phases 1 or 3 of the cleanse:
add more seeds and avocados to your meals.

The seeds will add protein and the fat from the avocados will burn slowly, extending the energy you get from each meal.

If you are in Phase 2 of the cleanse:
add protein to whichever Meal Option you are on.

Adding protein does not mean you are moving out of your Meal Option. You can be on the Transform Meal Option and add lean chicken to your mono-diet of kitchari without adding any of the foods from the other Meal Options. However, if you consistently feel like you need more blood sugar support, I recommend moving to the Rejuvenate or Nourish Meal Option until you feel stabilized.

4 Rehydration

Probably the most common cause of digestive problems, headaches, fatigue, lymph congestion and poor detoxification function is dehydration. Thus, one of our first priorities during the Colorado Cleanse is to deeply rehydrate all the cells of the body, especially the digestive tract.

Some of my patients are surprised when I tell them they are dehydrated. "But I drink tons of water," they protest. The fact is, it's possible to drink adequate amounts of water and still not drive that water deeply into the cells. You probably know the feeling of water going right through you. If this is occurring, we need to use some special techniques to make sure the body gets properly rehydrated.

During the Colorado Cleanse, we use two major techniques to rehydrate. I'll explain them both in detail in a moment, but first, here they are:

1. **Hot Sips:** Sip plain boiled hot water every 10 – 15 minutes throughout the day.

2. **Daily Ounces:** Drink ½ your ideal body weight in ounces of plain room-temperature water each day.

Hot Sips

Imagine pouring cold water on a dried out piece of leather. That water would most likely roll right down the leather, rather than soaking in. If the pores of the leather stay closed, the water molecules have no opportunity to penetrate.

A dried out digestive tract can experience the same effect. We may be drinking a lot of water, but if the intestinal wall doesn't have a chance to soften and become receptive to the water, rehydration may not occur.

Now imagine soaking the leather in hot water. You can just imagine how the pores would open up, allowing the water to penetrate and soften the material.

To create this softening, porous atmosphere, we sip boiled hot water throughout the day. This means 1-3 small sips every 10 – 15 minutes.

Sipping hot water is also a very effective and time-tested lymph-moving technique. By dilating the lymphatic channels, we make it much easier for the lymph to flow unobstructed, which is one of the main goals of the Colorado Cleanse.

Why boiled?

Bringing the water to a boil for a few seconds is a tenet of Ayurvedic hydration therapy, for several reasons. Boiling makes it easier to absorb into the cells. It also makes the water molecules very active, which is why boiled hot water is more cleansing than cold water.

Daily Ounces

Once your cells have been primed by the hot water, enter the water that will do the hydration legwork.

This is plain, room-temperature water, so it doesn't shock the pores closed again, as cold water might. We ask that you drink half your body weight in ounces each day, which is the best indicator I have found to address the hydration needs of most individuals. For example, if you ideally would weigh 140lbs, drink 70 ounces of water each day.

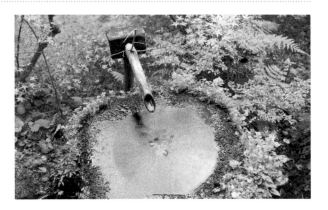

Why plain?

Cleansers always ask: "can I swap my water out for lemon water, herbal tea, juice, carbonated water, coconut water, rice milk, kombucha?"

Well, no, but not because we are trying to deprive you. Plain water has a rinsing effect that not even lemon water can replicate. Adding anything to water also creates an extra step for your body to achieve hydration: first it must separate the plain water molecule from whatever else it may be bound to, before it can drive that water deeply into the cell pores, called aquaporins.

So please, for the duration of this cleanse, make hydration as easy as possible for your body and follow the plain room-temperature water guideline, half your ideal body weight in ounces each day! I know it's a lot of water, so just do your best.

5 Herbs

*Note: If you are feeling discomfort during the cleanse, reduce or stop the herbs to pace the cleansing effects so they are a little more manageable for you.

Manjistha

Manjistha is a lymphatic de-stagnator and blood cleanser. In Ayurveda, the lymph is considered the first of the body tissues to become congested. Once the lymph is clogged, the other body tissues including blood, muscle, fat, bone, nerves and reproductive tissue, become congested in a kind of domino effect.

Most directly, lymph is responsible for immunity and the health of the skin, inside and out. Making sure the skin is properly drained into a healthy lymphatic system will determine how you look and feel.

Manjistha Dosage

- 400mg, 3 times per day, after each meal.
- If you tend to be sensitive to herbs take 1 capsule, 1-2 times per day after meals.
- LifeSpa's Manjistha formula contains Gokshura because it is a natural lymph and fluid regulator.
- Manjistha is a red root and, like beetroot, can turn your urine a slight reddish color. This is normal and nothing to be alarmed about.

Alternative to Manjistha: Try one dropperful of Red Root tincture in warm water after each meal.

Turmeric Plus

For thousands of years, this common spice was used in Ayurveda for muscle, joints, skin, mental clarity, intestinal health, bile flow and fat metabolism.

We use turmeric mainly to help support the intestinal villi. The villi are small, fingerlike projections that line the walls of our intestines, increasing the surface area so that we can absorb as many nutrients from our food as possible. They also play an important role in immunity and the removal of toxins.

Many factors - including overeating, rich and/or spicy food and coffee, yeast and unfriendly bacteria – can injure and irritate the intestinal villi. But perhaps the most pervasive reason for compromising the villi in our culture is stress.

When the villi are irritated, they usually become either too dry or bogged down by reactive mucus, which makes them nonfunctional.

Turmeric supports healthy intestinal villi and works to normalize the mucus on the intestinal wall and sinuses.

Turmeric Plus Dosage

- 500mg, 3 times per day, after each meal.
- If you tend to be sensitive to herbs take 1 capsule, 1–2 times per day after meals.
- LifeSpa's Turmeric Plus formula contains black pepper fruit, which in the proper ratio has been shown to increase the absorption of turmeric by 2000%!

Alternative to Turmeric Plus: Drink 1 cup of dandelion root tea after each meal. Or use a plain turmeric supplement 3 times per day, after each meal.

Liver Repair

All of our body systems are connected. The lymph, villi and liver should all work together to remove toxins. But when the lymph and villi don't pull their weight, the toxins get pushed back to the liver, and the liver gets overwhelmed.

When the liver gets overwhelmed, toxins spill back into the blood and eventually get stored in fatty tissue throughout the body and in the brain. Yikes!

A congested liver can also make the bile - which is responsible for our digestion of fats and emulsifying fat-soluble toxins - too thick, compromising our ability to digest rich foods like wheat, gluten, soy, dairy or fried foods, and meaning that the fat-soluble toxins never get properly processed.
Liver Repair is a combination of herbs that normalize liver function and support liver and gallbladder health.

Liver Repair Dosage

- 475mg, 3 times per day, after each meal.
- If you experience any loose stools or digestive discomfort, either stop or try taking just 1-2 capsules per day to find the dose that is best for you. Sometimes the liver flush can come on too quickly, which can cause loose stools.
- LifeSpa's Liver Repair formula contains organic Bhumyamalaki, wild harvested Barberry root Bark, organic Turmeric Root, organic Amalaki Fruit, and Guduchi Stem.

Alternative to Liver Repair: Take 250mg of Milk Thistle three times per day after food.

Beet Cleanse

Beet Cleanse is a unique formulation designed to support bile flow, thinning the bile and thereby helping de-stagnate the bile and pancreatic ducts.

Remember the thick bile that resulted from an overwhelmed liver? That thick bile can clog the bile and pancreatic ducts. The result can be a less-than-optimal ability to digest fats, and pancreatic enzymes that cannot flow freely into the small intestine, slowing down digestion overall.

De-congesting these ducts is not only crucial to increasing fat metabolism and resetting the body's natural detox process, it's also an important step in stabilizing blood sugar, energy and mood.

Beet Cleanse Dosage

- 500mg, 3 times per day, 15 minutes before meals.
- If you tend to be sensitive to herbs or have liver or gallbladder issues, start with 1 capsule per day.
- During Phase 3, you'll be taking increasing dosages of Beet Cleanse daily. These dosages are detailed in your Day-by-Day Guide on pages 18-31.
- LifeSpa's Beet Cleanse formula contains organic beet root, organic fenugreek seed, organic cinnamon bark and shilajit extract.

Alternative to Beet Cleanse: Eat more raw beets, 2-3 per day, and drink 1 cup of fenugreek tea after each meal. To make fenugreek tea, steep 1 tablespoon of fenugreek seed in 8 oz. of hot water for 20 minutes.

Regenerate

Whether we know it or not, many of us are deeply exhausted from our go go go, mind-over-matter lifestyle in a culture that glorifies stress. When we come into a powerful cleanse experience such as the Colorado Cleanse, we give our nervous system the opportunity to unwind. But after being held in a pattern of continuous stress and exhaustion, it often takes a little coaxing to help the nervous system to feel safe enough to experience peace and calm.

Regenerate is a formula based on the super-herb Shilajit, which is actually a resin rather than an herb. Shilajit is one of the most amazing "herbs" for deep rejuvenation, and has been used for millennia to support:

- Energy
- Balanced mood
- Memory
- Absorption and efficacy of nutrients
- Mental clarity
- Blood sugar levels
- Natural detox processes of the body
- Optimal oxygenation of the cells

Regenerate Dosage

- 300mg, 3 times per day, after each meal.
- If you tend to be sensitive to herbs, start with 1 capsule per day.
- To maximize the benefits of Shilajit, LifeSpa's Regenerate formula uses the ancient combination of Shilajit, Ashwagandha and Amalaki - considered to be synergistic herbs - in traditional Ayurvedic proportions.

Alternatives to Shilajit: Shilajit is a rare herb and hard to replace. Adaptogens like American Ginseng or Astragalus can provide excellent rejuvenation, though many of the other benefits of Shilajit will go unmatched.

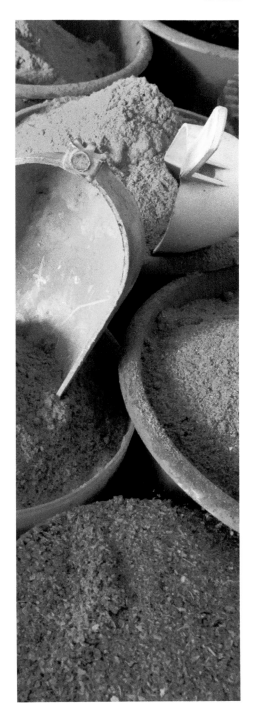

Sugar Destroyer

For years, before cleansers embark on our Group Colorado Cleanse, we have been asking them to take a survey reporting their symptoms and areas of concern. Cravings are one of the most common issues reported. In fact, they are epidemic in our culture. Whether it's coffee, chips or dark chocolate in the afternoon, cravings are usually an indication of imbalance in the blood sugar.

LifeSpa's Sugar Destroyer is an herbal formula built around Gymnema sylvestre, an Ayurvedic herb that has classically been used to slow the absorption of sugar through the taste buds and intestinal wall into the bloodstream. When sugar absorption is slowed, cravings are reduced and the body is given an opportunity to restore balance in the blood sugar, bringing us one step closer to proper fat metabolism!

> Note: Even if you don't have symptoms of blood sugar imbalance, this protocol is important to decongest the pancreatic duct and support healthy blood sugar levels during the Colorado Cleanse.

Sugar Destroyer Dosage

- 500mg, 3 times per day, 15 minutes before meals.
- If you tend to be sensitive to herbs, start with 1 capsule per day.
- LifeSpa's Sugar Destroyer formula combines Gymnema sylvestre with Shilajit to optimize efficacy.

Alternative to Sugar Destroyer: Cinnamon tea – steep a cinnamon stick in hot water for 20 minutes and drink 1 cup 15 minutes before each meal.

Warm or Cool Digest

An overwhelming majority of us have less-than-optimal digestion. Ideally, the digestion is strong enough to process most anything in reasonable amounts and in moderation, and to absorb a large amount of nutrition from modest amounts of food.

Cravings, overeating, gas, bloating, intestinal discomfort, and occasional heartburn are all possible signs of compromised digestion, among others.

In my practice, I have found two major styles of digestive imbalance. The first is a weak "digestive fire," or agni, as it is called in Ayurveda. Ayurveda, as well as Chinese, Tibetan and other forms of traditional medicine, view the digestive system as a fire that needs to be strong enough to digest or "cook" the food we have ingested and then assimilate its nutrients. When this fire is weak, we get what I refer to as boggy digestion – too little hydrochloric acid (HCL), resulting in undigested food, gas, bloating, and feelings of heaviness and fatigue.

To address this style of imbalance, we use an herbal formulation called Warm Digest. Warm Digest is a traditional combination of the herbs pippali, ginger and black pepper that warms the belly and stokes the digestive fire.

The second major style of digestive imbalance is an overly acidic digestion. Too much HCL acid can result in occasional acid digestion (occasional heartburn).

To address this, we use the herbal formulation Cool Digest, a blend of Ayurvedic herbs to cool and soothe a hot and irritated digestive tract while simultaneously strengthening the digestive function.

LifeSpa's Cool Digest formula is a blend of organic Avipattikar Churna formula, organic Amalaki, organic Guduchi, and Asafoetida Resin (Hing).

Warm or Cool Digest Dosage

- 450-500mg of Warm Digest or Cool Digest, 3 times per day, 15 minutes before meals with 12 oz. of water.
- If you tend to be sensitive to herbs, start with 1 capsule per day.
- During Phase 3, you'll be taking increasing dosages of Warm or Cool Digest daily. These dosages are detailed in your Day-by-Day Guide on pages 18-31.

Alternatives to Warm Digest: Make what I call "Ginger Pizzas": slice fresh, raw, peeled ginger root into thin rounds. Sprinkle with lemon juice and sea salt. Chew 2 of these 15 minutes before each meal, and store in the fridge for up to 2 days.

Alternative to Cool Digest: Stir a pinch of ginger, cumin and fennel powders into one cup of hot water. Drink with each meal.

6 12-Minute Workout

During the Colorado Cleanse, we are working towards fat metabolism – the ability of the body to burn fat as its fuel. This is also the goal of proper exercise, and when it lines up, exercise helps us to naturally lose weight, detoxify, boost energy, and stabilize our mood.

I find that, when it comes to exercise, many of us tend to do too much. If we drive the body to the point of exhaustion, at some point our progress plateaus, and we can experience a lot of discouragement as a result. In my first book, *Body, Mind, and Sport*, I shared my story of being an exhausted and frustrated triathlete and how, only when I began to train less and rest more, did I begin to progress again.

The 12-Minute Workout is based on the principles of heart rate variability - which aims to strengthen the heart by increasing the difference between the resting heart rate and maximum heart rate during exercise – and a principle I call "chasing the rabbit," which mimics the fitness achieved in a hunter-gatherer situation, when exercise was part of survival.

Over the next two weeks, I urge you to use the 12-Minute Workout as a simple, versatile and doable form of exercise program. You may love it. During the cleanse, use this as a cardiovascular base, and avoid pushing with too much other cardio. After the cleanse, you can use this as your entire workout or as a cardiovascular warm-up before yoga, a bike ride or hiking.

If you don't yet have an established exercise routine, the 12-Minute Workout is a fabulous start.

Here are some of the benefits:

- Increase fat metabolism
- Calm the nervous system and mind
- Support healthy glucose and insulin levels
- Increase calorie burning
- Boost energy
- Create a sleeker, stronger, and more toned physique
- Enhance sex drive
- Improve lymphatic drainage, leading to healthier skin and detoxification
- Amplify exercise endurance and performance
- Raise human growth hormone – which may be responsible for all of the above

12-Minute Workout

Sprint Recovery Training

First, choose a form of cardiovascular exercise to practice using the 12-Minute Workout prompts below. This can be walking, jogging, riding a bike or using a cardio machine. It can also be jumping jacks, running up and down stairs, jumping on and off a curb. For the elderly or those who cannot use their legs, I have recommended lifting soup cans in the past. You can get creative here - anything that will get your heart rate up. The entire 12-Minute Workout is done breathing through the nose.

12-Minute Workout	Min.	Activity
Step 1: Warm Up Exercise slowly for 2 minutes while breathing deeply in and out through your nose.	1	Warm Up
	2	
Step 2: Sprint Start exercising faster, like a mini sprint, for 1 minute. Using the nasal breath during the sprint will keep you from overexerting yourself. Don't push it here. Start slow and build yourself up to a faster sprint over time. Try to do a sprint pace that you can maintain for one minute. In a couple of weeks, you'll be sprinting like a pro.	3	Sprint
	4	Recovery
Step 3: Recovery Slow the exercise down to the warm-up pace for one minute, maintaining the nasal breathing if you can.	5	Sprint
Step 4: Second Sprint Start another sprint for one minute. Make this a little faster than the first sprint if you can.	6	Recovery
	7	Sprint
Step 5: Second Recovery Recover from the sprint with one minute of deep nasal breathing at the warm up pace. If you cannot maintain nasal breathing during the recovery, it's an indication that the sprint was too hard. With each sprint, it will get easier.	8	Recovery
	9	Sprint
Step 6: Continue Sprints and Recoveries Continue sprints and recoveries for a total of 4 sprints and 4 recoveries. Follow the nasal breathing if you can.	10	Recovery
Step 7: Cool Down Repeat Step 1. Exercise at the warm up pace, gradually slowing down, for 2 minutes.	11	Cool Down
	12	

Note: In the beginning you may need 90 seconds of recovery rather than just one minute. If this is the case, do the 2 minute warm up followed by 3 rounds of sprints and recoveries rather than 4, making the recoveries 90 seconds each. Include a 2.5 minute cool down. Your workout will still come to 12 minutes.

Most of all, nasal breathing makes it possible for us to be calm and exercise at the same time! Athletes call this "the zone." Using this technique, many have found that a workout doesn't have to feel like hard work after all.

During the rest and recovery phases, nasal breathing forces air into the lower lobes of the lungs allowing for more efficient release of CO_2, not to mention activation of the calming rest-and-digest parasympathetic nervous system that is accessible through the lower lobes of the lungs. This will help you release toxins and stress.

Breathing through your nose during this or any workout has multiple benefits. For one, nasal breathing helps us gauge how much is too much. We know that we are overexerting ourselves when nasal breathing becomes impossible and we have to gasp for air through our mouths.

Nasal breathing is a skill that may take some time to master. Don't worry if at first you have to breathe through your mouth. Do the best you can and, in time, nasal breathing will become easier and feel more natural.

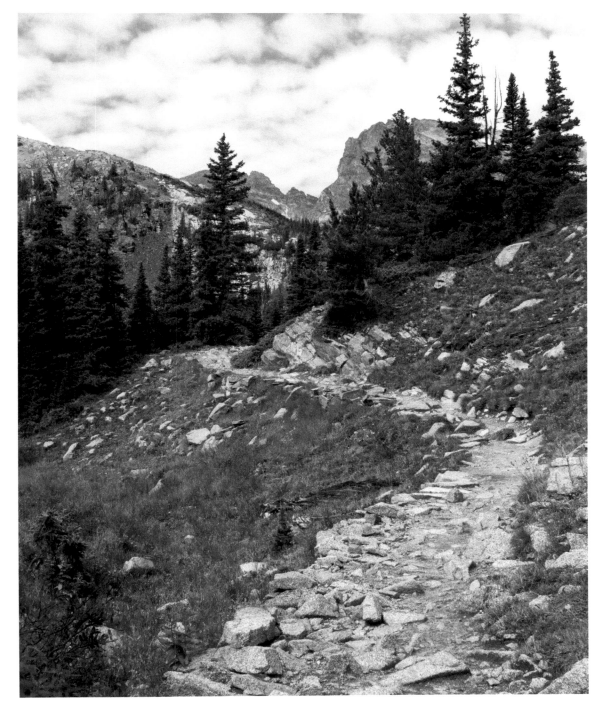

7

Optional Stress-Relief Practices

In this chapter, I'll give you some time-tested lifestyle practices that can transform the Colorado Cleanse from a very powerful experience to a potentially life-changing one.

One of the biggest draws of a cleanse is the shift in mental and spiritual clarity many experience when their bodies are detoxing. As our bodies begin to let go of toxins – or what Ayurveda calls ama – we are given an opportunity to find deep stillness within. Practices that encourage calm and stillness, such as the ones in this chapter, may feel easier and more fruitful when you are cleansing.

These practices also help the lymphatic system release toxins more effectively, which can help to soothe detox-related body aches and pains.

You can choose which of these practices is realistic for you during the Colorado Cleanse, but I strongly encourage you to commit to the ones you can fit in and do them consistently.

Here they are:

- Yoga – Sun Salutations
- Breathing Exercises (Pranayama)
- Meditation
- Abhyanga Self-Massage

All of these practices are discussed in detail and demonstrated on my Gaiam DVD *Ayurveda for Detox.*

Yoga – Sun Salutations

Called *Surya Namaskara* in Sanskrit, Sun Salutations are a series of twelve *asanas*, or poses, performed in a fluid sequence. Done properly, they:

* strengthen and stretch all the major muscle groups
* lubricate the joints
* condition the spine
* massage the internal organs
* increase blood flow and circulation

Surya Namaskara (Sun Salutations)

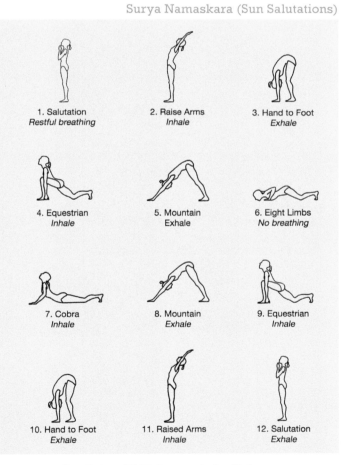

1. Salutation
Restful breathing

2. Raise Arms
Inhale

3. Hand to Foot
Exhale

4. Equestrian
Inhale

5. Mountain
Exhale

6. Eight Limbs
No breathing

7. Cobra
Inhale

8. Mountain
Exhale

9. Equestrian
Inhale

10. Hand to Foot
Exhale

11. Raised Arms
Inhale

12. Salutation
Exhale

Synchronizing the movements with the breath helps to activate prana, or life force. During the Colorado Cleanse, we emphasize this even more by holding each pose for 1-2 minutes while breathing deeply through your nose. If you are new to yoga, start slowly and be gentle with your ability. You do not need to do the poses perfectly to benefit.

Doing 1 – 3 Sun Salutations in the morning to wake up your body and get the prana flowing is a powerful way to get the most out of the Colorado Cleanse.

You can also follow my Everyday Yoga program on the Gaiam DVD *Ayurveda for Detox.*

Breathing Exercises – Pranayama

Pranayama means "extension of the breath," or "extension of the life force," and it refers to a class of breathing exercises that originate in the yogic tradition. These exercises are meant to control the flow of prana to bring it back into a balanced state.

Different forms of pranayama have different effects and are done for different purposes. Here are three pranayama exercises that can be done in sequence for a well-rounded and balancing experience, or on their own for more targeted effects:

Ujjayi Pranayama *(pronounced oo-jai)***:**
Grounding; Purifying; Calms and Focuses the Mind

- Start in a comfortable seated position.

- Inhale slowly, then, holding your palm about six inches in front of your mouth, open your mouth and exhale through your mouth onto your palm as if you are trying to fog up a mirror. Notice the constriction in the back of your throat that naturally occurs when you breathe like this.

- Now, replicate that same constriction in your throat while inhaling and exhaling deeply through the nose with your mouth closed.

- Bring your attention to how smooth the breath feels here, as though it is a golden thread that you are pulling with control over the back of your throat.

- Inhale for 4 counts, exhale for 4 counts.

- Try breathing like this for this for 2 – 5 minutes, 1-2 times per day.

- This breath can be more calming (yin) or more activating (yang) depending on how forcefully you breathe. More forceful breathing would be more activating and vice versa.

Nadi Shodhana *(Alternate Nostril Breathing – pronounced nah-dee sho-dah-nah)*:
Balancing; Brings Composure and Calm by Oxygenating Both Sides of the Brain

- Start in a comfortable seated position.

- With your right hand, take either your thumb and middle finger or thumb and ring finger – whichever is more comfortable – to either sides of your nose, so that both fingers are ready to close a nostril.

- First, gently close your left nostril and inhale through your right nostril.

- Next, switch the plug and exhale through your left nostril with the right nostril closed.

- Inhale through the same nostril – the left – with your right nostril still closed.

- Switch the plug and exhale through your right nostril with the left nostril closed.

- Long, slow inhalations and exhalations are more relaxing, while shorter inhalations and exhalations are more energizing.

- Repeat this cycle for 5 -10 minutes, 1-2 times per day.

Meditation

Meditation is a powerful way to anchor into stillness and take that experience with you into your day. Before we start a meditation practice, often we are not even aware of how busy our minds are. During the Colorado Cleanse, we get a special opportunity to quiet our minds because we eliminate the stimulating nature of many foods, including caffeine, sugar and alcohol, and encourage fat metabolism, which is by nature stabilizing.

If you already have a meditation practice that works well for you, please continue. If not, you can begin with my One-Minute Meditation, which I will describe below. This technique can be used on its own for literally a minute, or as part of a longer meditation.

One-Minute Meditation

The One-Minute Meditation consists of two parts – 30 seconds of bellows breathing followed by 30 seconds of stillness.

Bellows Breathing:
With your eyes closed, breathe deeply through your nose, in and out, using all five lobes of your lungs as if they were a big bellows. In other words, inhale and exhale as deeply and as quickly as possible, within your comfort range. If you feel dizzy, stop!
Driving breath into the lower lobes of your lungs this way stimulates the calming, parasympathetic nervous system.

Stillness:
Follow the bellows breath with 30 seconds – or longer – of silent stillness with the eyes closed. When thoughts resurface, use another round of bellows breath for 10-20 seconds to oxygenate the brain and settle the mind.

Longer Meditation: 10 – 20 minutes
Follow the instructions for the One-Minute Meditation, and then sit in stillness in a comfortable seated position. When you notice thoughts arise, do 8-10 bellows breaths to infuse the mind with stillness. Don't worry if this seems painfully frequent – when you begin to work with the mind, it can be shocking to see how busy our minds are. Commit to regarding yourself and your practice with compassion no matter what arises.

Abhyanga Self-Massage

Daily self-massage, called *Abhyanga*, is a powerful way to calm and disarm the nervous system while activating detoxification pathways. Traditionally, herb-infused sesame oil is used to lubricate the skin and coat the nervous system with a soothing and protective layer against the elements. This allows us to walk through our days more centered and calm. Other benefits include:

- Lubricate and promote flexibility of the muscles, tissues, and joints
- Promote softness, youthfulness and luster of the skin

    Don't underestimate the power of Abhyanga!

Preparation:

First, you'll need a massage oil. You can use plain sesame, olive or coconut oil, or you can purchase a herb-infused massage oil such as LifeSpa's *Lymphatic Massage Oil,* a blend formulated specifically for moving the lymph. Herbalized oils will provide better moisturizing for the skin and under-skin layer than plain oil, which sometimes can cause dryness.

Curing the oil

Traditionally, oil is purified before being applied to the skin with a simple process called "curing." This changes the molecular structure of the oil, enabling your skin to absorb it better. You can cure your oil by heating it to about 220 degrees Fahrenheit.

Here's a neat tip: 220 degrees is the boiling point of water at sea level. By adding a few drops of water to your oil in the beginning, you'll know you've reached the proper temperature when the water starts to boil and evaporate.

LifeSpa's Lymphatic and Tri-Doshic Massage Oils have already been cured for you, eliminating this step.

Safety note: Since oils are flammable, they should:

- Always be cured slowly on low heat.
- Never left unattended.
- Once the oil reaches the proper temperature, remove it from the heat and store in a safe place to cool gradually.

Once your oil is ready, you're all set for Abhyanga.

Here's how it's done:

Heat ¼ cup of cured oil to slightly above body temperature. If you have a pre-purchased bottle of massage oil, you can simply place the bottle in a cup or bowl of warm water for a few minutes.
If time permits, follow the procedure below before getting in the shower. If time does not permit, you can do a quick version in the shower. Some people actually prefer to do Abhyanga in the shower. Not only do the warm water and steam help the oil absorb into your skin, the water helps a small amount of oil spread evenly over a large area of skin. Thus, you can use less oil and rinse off lightly afterwards (no scrubbing) to remove excess oil.

Note: The entire Abhyanga massage should be with the palm of the hand rather than with the fingertips.

1. Head Massage:

Start by massaging your head. Place a small amount of oil on your palms and begin to massage the scalp vigorously with the palm of your hand. The head and the feet are considered the most important parts of the body to massage, so really take some time here.

2. Face and Ears:

With the open part of the hand, gently apply oil to your face and outer ears.

3 Neck:

Massage both the front and back of your neck, and the upper part of the spine. Continue to use your open hand in a rubbing type of motion.

4. Body Application:

Apply a small amount of oil to your entire body before proceeding to massage each area of the body. This has the added benefit of letting the oil have more time in contact with your skin.

5. Arms, Hands and Fingers:

Massage your arms. The ideal motion is back and forth over your long bones, and circular movements over your joints. Massage both arms, including the hands and fingers.

6. Chest and Abdomen:

A very gentle circular motion should be used over your heart. Over your abdomen, use a gentle circular motion following the bowel pattern. In other words, moving clockwise from the right lower part of the abdomen up towards the right upper part of the abdomen, over to the upper left, down to the lower left, then over to the lower right (down on the left, up on the right).

7. Back and Spine:

Massage your back and spine. There will be some areas which you may have difficulty reaching. Do the best you can – or ask your partner for help.

8. Legs:

Massage your legs. Like the arms, use a back and forth motion over the long bones and a circular motion over the joints.

9. Feet:

Lastly, massage the bottom of the feet. The feet are considered especially important, so give them some extra time. Use the open part of your hand and massage vigorously back and forth over the soles of the feet.

Enjoy these potent practices for finding peace and stillness during the Colorado Cleanse, and for the rest of your life!

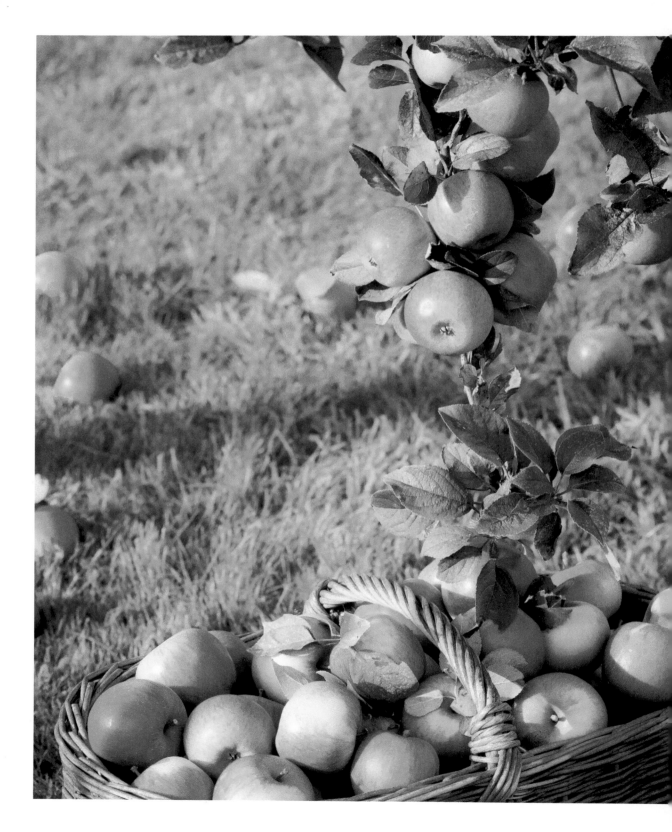

Phase 1
Pre-Cleanse

Apples
Beet Tonic
Green Tonic

8 Apples

Some of our main allies in thinning the bile and detoxing the gut wall during Phase 1 are apples. This is achieved by two potent ingredients in apples: malic acid and pectin:

- **Malic acid** not only thins the bile, it actually helps dilate the bile ducts and the liver's biliary tubes, which will be used as pathways for detoxification in this cleanse as well as in daily life when we reset your body's ability to detox naturally and constantly.

- **Apple pectin** is a great detoxifier of the intestinal villi and the gut wall.

During Phase 1, give yourself the permission to eat a whole lot more apples than you normally may. Apples have been hybridized to be very sweet. Originally, they were sour and tart. The more sour the apple, the more malic acid it contains. The goal is 3 - 5 organic, non-GMO apples per day.

While Ayurveda recommends spacing fruit consumption apart from that of other foods for reasons of digestive ease, apples are an exception. During Phase 1 and 3 of the Colorado Cleanse they can be eaten directly after a meal. In the case of a blood sugar crash, an apple can be eaten alone as a balancing snack.

Make the apples part of your meals.

Exception: in the case of a blood sugar crash, when you find yourself needing a snack to balance blood sugar, an apple is a good choice. Make a note to eat more protein at your next meal (see Blood Sugar Balancing on page 36 for tips on adding protein to meals).
If you have unstable blood sugar: Stick with tart green apples rather than the sweeter red or yellow varieties. This will cut down the sugar content significantly. If you can't have apples at all, use malic acid powder instead (see Malic Acid Protocol below).

Malic Acid Protocol*
(If you prefer not to eat apples)

Stir 1-2 teaspoons into 8 oz. of water and drink up to three times daily.

*Malic Acid Powder is available from LifeSpa's online store, as well as the supplement section of some natural health food stores. Though a great bile thinner and replacement for apples during the Colorado Cleanse, Malic Acid powder is very tart! Don't say we didn't warn you.

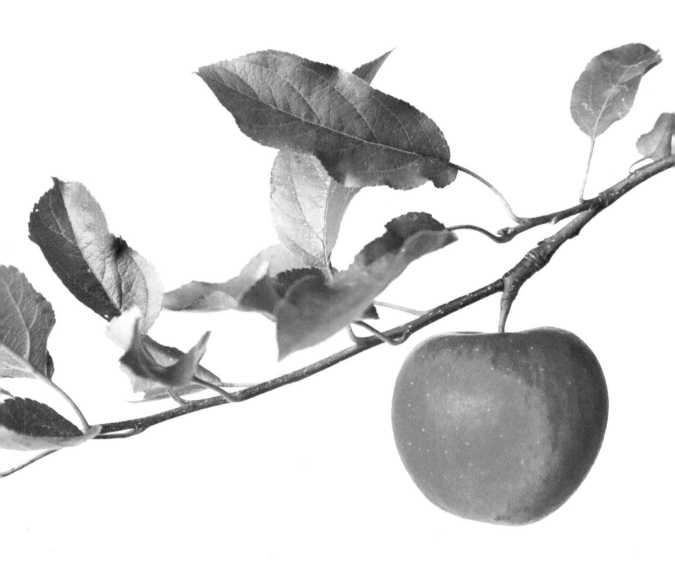

9 Beet Tonic

Your diet for Phase 1 of the cleanse will include more beets than you may be used to. During Phase 1, we are honing in on a high-fiber diet that will scrub the intestinal villi of any congestion that may have built up over time. We are also working on thinning the bile, which will contribute to stronger digestion and natural detoxification in the long run.

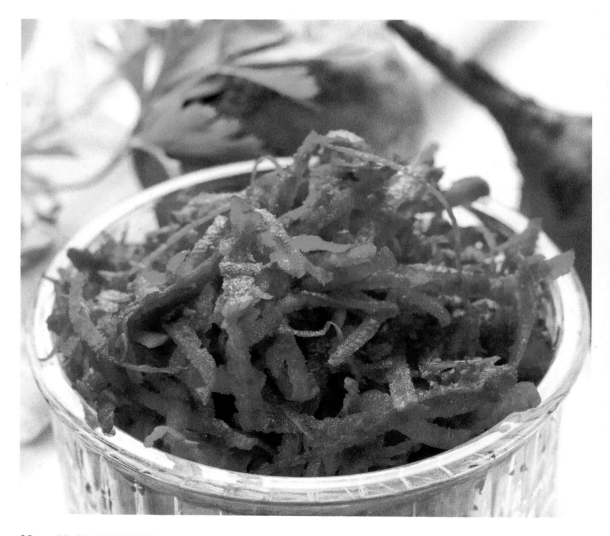

In addition to being some of the best bile-thinning agents known, beets – like other red roots - are lymph movers. That's two of the key goals of the Colorado Cleanse covered in one sweet, easy-to-find root.

During the four days of Phase 1, I will ask you to eat 1-2 raw beets each day with meals. While cooked or roasted beets still offer some of the benefits, it is raw beets that really pack the punch. Try the Beet Tonic recipe below to dress up your raw beets the Colorado Cleanse way and reap all the benefits.

Beet Tonic

Makes 1 serving (depending on beet size)

Ingredients:

1 raw beet, peeled and grated
The juice of half a lemon
Dijon mustard and fresh ginger root (optional)

Method:
Combine all ingredients and eat immediately or save covered in the fridge for up to 24 hours. The Beet Tonic can be eaten as a side dish or topping to an entrée, soup, or steamed or raw veggies.

10 Green Tonic

This is the second "tonic" you will make friends with in Phase 1 of this cleanse. It's something between a soup and a smoothie.

The purpose of the Green Tonic is to rejuvenate the bile and liver. It's chock-full of vital nutrients that are made accessible via the steaming and blending of the vegetables, which helps to break down the cell wall.

I'll ask you to have 1–2 (8 oz.) servings of the Green Tonic each day, with meals.

Green Tonic

Makes about 2 (8 oz.) servings

Ingredients:

1-2 cups filtered water for steaming
2 medium celery stalks, chopped
1 whole zucchini, chopped
1 cup string beans, ends trimmed and chopped
½ cup fresh parsley

Method:

Steam all the vegetables except parsley for about 8 minutes or until bright green, tender but not mushy (try not to overcook, as over-cooking can start to decrease nutrient value).

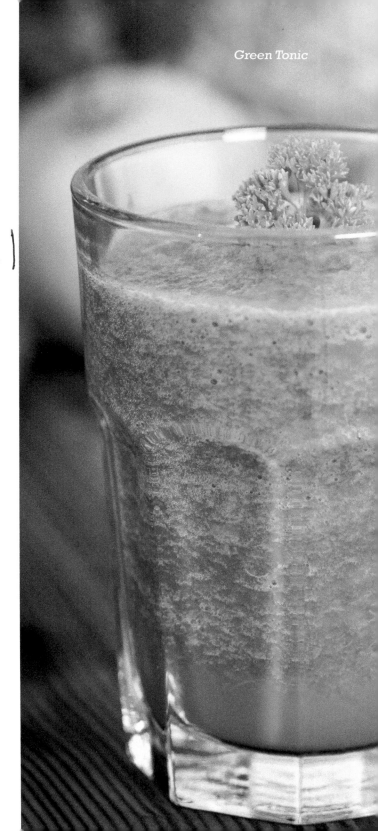

Combine all the ingredients, including the fresh parsley, in a blender using the remaining steaming water as a thinning agent. Puree until smooth, adding more water as needed to reach your desired consistency. If you have a Vitamix or a similarly powerful blender, you can make the Green Tonic very smooth. A weaker blender or food processor may result in a chunkier, less unified texture.

To support digestion, please drink the Green Tonic at room temperature, warm, or hot – not cold.

Flavor Options:

Green Tonic Soup (Warm and Savory):

Make it a "soup" by adding garlic, ginger, salt and pepper to taste. Serve warm with a squeeze of lemon.

Green Tonic Smoothie:

Add 1 small beet with a slice of fresh ginger and the juice of ½ a lemon.

* While the above recipe is recommended, if you need variety you may use any of the greens from the appropriate Seasonal Cleansing Foods list in Appendix 2 of this book.

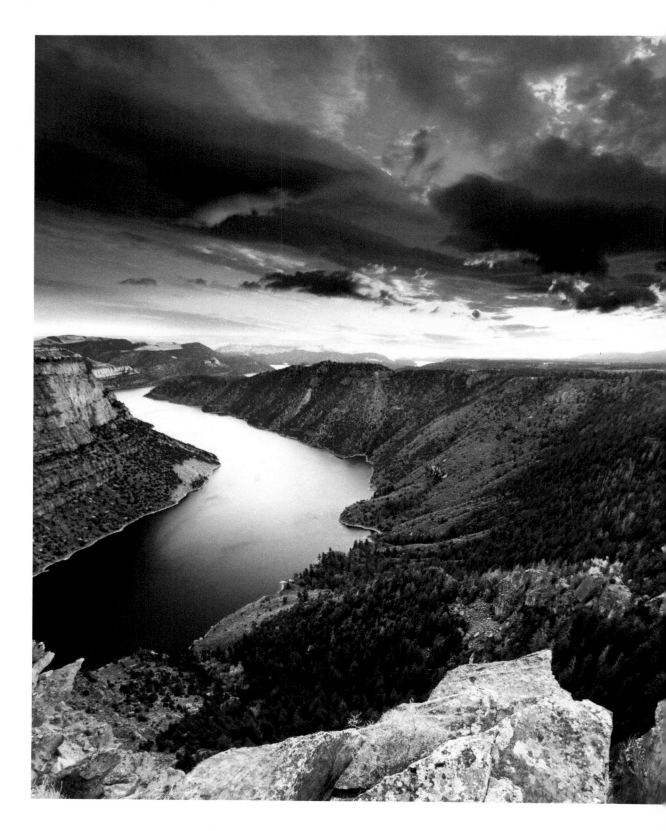

Phase 2
Main Cleanse

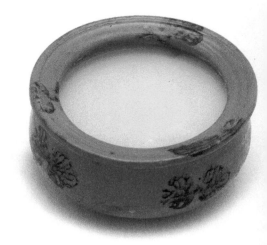

11 Morning Ghee

What is Ghee?

Ghee is a golden-colored, heat-stable oil that is made by separating the fat particles of milk from the water, milk solids, lactose, and impurities via the natural process of simmering. A kind of clarified butter, ghee has been revered in Ayurveda as a healing, universally-balancing oil for thousands of years.

The Purpose of Morning Ghee

During Phase 2, you will take increasing doses of ghee first thing every morning. In Ayurveda, this process is called oleation *(snehana)*. Only follow the advanced ghee dosages if you have successfully completed the cleanse before and tolerated the ghee well.

Oleation has several purposes:

- Delivers fat-soluble nutrients during the cleanse
- Bonds to fat-soluble toxins and drives them to the colon for elimination
- Deeply and thoroughly lubricates all the body's tissues from the inside out
- Triggers fat metabolism
- Gently flushes the liver and gallbladder

Triggering fat metabolism is key during this cleanse. Imagine this: the ghee enters your body and binds to fat-soluble toxins – which are the pesky toxins that stay lodged in the fat cells in our bodies, usually for decades. Once the toxins are bound, burning those toxin-containing fat cells through fat metabolism means that you are initiating the detox process right away.

Morning Ghee	
Day	Teaspoons of Ghee
5	2 tsp
6	4 tsp
7	4 tsp
8	6 tsp
9	8 tsp
10	8 tsp
11	10 tsp

Once fat burning begins, you will:

- Experience the calm, stable, mood-balancing effects of this fuel that our bodies were designed to run on.
- Support bile and lymph flow which are dependent on fat metabolism.
- Have greater endurance as fat is the endurance fuel.
- Burn calm fuel that slowly disarms the protective nervous system and moves toxic mental and emotional patterns.
- Recalibrate healthy blood sugar levels.
- Release fat-soluble toxins.

Why Ghee?

While ghee has been the traditional and preferred oil for oleation, you can use other oils. If needed, the alternatives we recommend are flax seed oil and olive oil. **If you do not have a gallbladder,** coconut oil may be a good option as it does not flush the liver and gallbladder the same way the other oils do.

The major reasons to not use ghee are if you are vegan or have a strong reaction to the taste. Most people who are lactose intolerant do not experience an intolerance reaction to ghee, as it has been stripped of all lactose.

Advanced Ghee Dosages	
Day	Teaspoons of Ghee
5	3 tsp
6	6 tsp
7	9 tsp
8	12 tsp
9	15 tsp
10	18 tsp
11	21 tsp

Maintain a Nonfat Diet During Oleation

In order to achieve the benefits of oleation, the Morning Ghee protocol must be paired with a nonfat diet. For the seven-day period of Phase 2, your only fat intake will be the Morning Ghee, which will trigger fat metabolism during the day as long as the diet remains fat-free.

Keep Your Bowels Moving

During Phase 2, as the toxins are building up in the gut, it is essential to maintain regular bowel movements (see page 142 of the FAQ section for help with constipation). Morning Ghee may loosen stools in some people. As long as you are not experiencing discomfort, this is fine and you can continue increasing the Morning Ghee as planned.

When to Back Off on Ghee

You may need to reduce the ghee dosage if you are:

- Experiencing strong muscle aches and pains
- Dealing with lingering nausea (mild nausea can be quelled by sipping hot water, ginger tea, or eating a meal)
- Losing weight too quickly
- Feeling general malaise that is inhibiting your ability to function adequately

These are signs that the detox process is moving too quickly. No worries – we can slow it down to a comfortable pace.

The first thing to do is to stop the herbs (see top of page 40 for more on this).

The second thing to do is to reduce the ghee dosages and go back to the dosage at which you felt comfortable. Even if you have to stay at 2–3 teaspoons of ghee during Phase 2, you will still be getting the benefits, as the ghee will be attracting toxins and depositing them into the intestinal tract.

The third thing to do is to eat off the Nourish meal plan and add protein if necessary (see Blood Sugar Balancing on page 36).

12 Meal Options

One of the best things about the Colorado Cleanse is the variety of nourishing meal options available to you while maintaining an effective detox.

We all enter this cleanse from where we are, which varies from person to person. In the many years of leading thousands of people through the Colorado Cleanse, I have observed that most of us want to try the most challenging option first. Resist this urge. Or, examine this urge for what it is: a noble intention that, for the purposes of this cleanse, could actually undermine your results by creating unnecessary stress. Stress will prevent your body from entering fat burning mode and properly balancing blood sugar, two key goals of this cleanse.

Here I've listed the Meal Options from the most inclusive, most doable plan, to the most austere plan, deliberately in that order because – unless you have done the Colorado Cleanse before and have a good sense of your digestive strength and the state of your blood sugar – the first option is where I would like you to begin. If you find it very easy, you are welcome to move to the next Meal Option. Do so mindfully; listen to your body every step of the way and back off if you experience discomfort.

Remember, the golden rule during Phase 2 is a nonfat diet.

*You can bounce back and forth between meal options each day, or even each meal, as needed.

What is Discomfort?

When I talk about discomfort in the Colorado Cleanse, I mean to differentiate between two styles of discomfort:

- The good kind: sometimes, a little discipline is good. Change is often perceived as discomfort, as when we kick a habit or addiction. We may feel generally healthier and even have more energy, but there is discomfort because we are used to living in a different state. If you experience this style of discomfort during the cleanse, experiment by sticking with the Meal Option you are on and being present with the discomfort. Remember that it's normal to feel a little more tired and sensitive. There are usually great gifts to be gleaned on the other side.

- The bad kind: Insidiously, we can cross over into pushing our bodies at the will of our minds. If your body is straining, please back off. Why? Because one of the worst and ultimately most discouraging things that can happen on this cleanse is a blood sugar crash – when our blood sugar dips too low, we are prone to binge eating, blowing up at our kids or spouses, or doing something else that can stress us out and undermine the cleanse benefits.

Differentiating between these two styles will take some tuning into your body. Stick with it. This is a great tool to develop for the rest of your life.

Meal Option 3: Nourish

Most Stabilizing to Blood Sugar Levels or a Busy/Active Lifestyle
Kitchari + Steamed Veggies + Salad + Oatmeal

This is the gentlest, most nourishing meal option that will still take you in the direction of balancing your blood sugar without risking a blood sugar crash. The main key is to avoid fat during the entire cleanse, which you will be doing. You will still benefit from a thorough detox on the Nourish meal option.

Kitchari: The staple of this meal option, like the other options, is kitchari.* Kitchari is a combination of split yellow mung beans and white basmati rice. Both have their husks removed to make them easier to digest (like baby food), and to heal your gut during Phase 2. The combination is a perfect protein and therefore keeps the blood sugar stable. See Chapter 1 – "What You'll Need" – for sources of kitchari and kitchari ingredients.*

In addition to kitchari, you can eat the following:

Steamed Veggies: Any veggies off the appropriate Seasonal Cleansing Foods list in Appendix 2 of this book.

Fruit: Cooked or raw seasonal fruit can be a meal on its own (ideally breakfast), and raw seasonal fruit, especially apples, make a good snack if you feel your blood sugar is crashing and you absolutely need something to get you to the next meal. Choose fruit with a low glycemic index (see page 118 for a note on fruit).

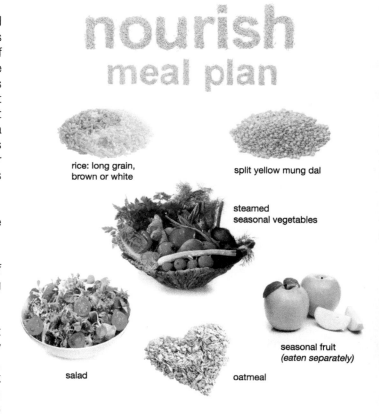

nourish
meal plan

rice: long grain, brown or white

split yellow mung dal

steamed seasonal vegetables

seasonal fruit (eaten separately)

salad

oatmeal

Salad: Raw seasonal greens and veggies.

Oatmeal: Remember not to add any fat or sweeteners!

Optional: If the taste of kitchari is not working for you, you can substitute any gluten-free grain with beans. Small beans are easier to digest than large beans.

If Your Blood Sugar Crashes

You may need to add more protein to your meals to keep your blood sugar stable. Have a nonfat snack such as an apple and plan to eat more protein at your next meal. See Blood Sugar Balancing on page 36 for more on adding protein. Remember that it can take a few weeks to balance blood sugar, and it's okay if you need to have a snack between meals in the beginning.

*You can bounce back and forth between meal options each day, or even each meal, as needed.

Meal Option 2: Rejuvenate

A Little Extra Support for Fragile Blood Sugar
Kitchari + Steamed Veggies

The Rejuvenate meal option is the middle road. It's a perfect place to start if you've done the cleanse before and want to ease in, and a great backup to jump to if you have a busy day or need a little more nourishment at a given meal. You can also transition from Nourish to Rejuvenate if you are feeling good and want a bit more of a challenge.

Kitchari: The staple. See Chapter 1 – "What You'll Need" – for sources of kitchari and kitchari ingredients.*

Steamed Veggies: Any veggies off the appropriate Seasonal Cleansing Foods list in Appendix 2 of this book can be steamed and added to your kitchari or served on the side.

Optional: If the taste of kitchari is not working for you, you can substitute any gluten-free grain with beans. Small beans are easier to digest than large beans.

If Your Blood Sugar Crashes

You may need to add more protein to your meals to keep your blood sugar stable. Have a nonfat snack such as an apple and plan to eat more protein at your next meal. See Blood Sugar Balancing on page 36 for more on adding protein. Remember that it can take a few weeks to balance blood sugar, and it's okay if you need to have a snack between meals in the beginning.

*You can bounce back and forth between meal options each day, or even each meal, as needed.

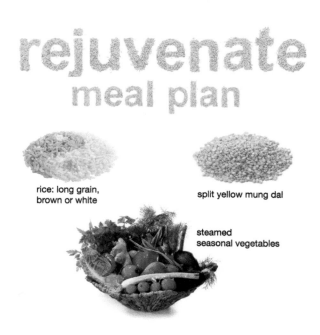

rejuvenate meal plan

rice: long grain, brown or white

split yellow mung dal

steamed seasonal vegetables

Meal Option 1: Transform

Most Detoxifying and Healing
Kitchari

If your blood sugar and digestion are strong enough, you may try eating a mono-diet of nonfat kitchari. If you are ready for it, this will be incredibly healing to your digestive tract and extremely detoxifying. When you eat a mono-diet, your body can focus the energy normally spent on digestion on cleansing and healing other systems.

Kitchari: The staple. See Chapter 1 – "What You'll Need" – for sources of kitchari and kitchari ingredients.*

In addition, follow these Transform meal guidelines:

Always eat your largest serving of kitchari midday when your digestion is the strongest. For dinner, eat early and eat a small serving with some warm water or herbal tea.

On this meal plan you can eat 3-4 meals per day to keep your blood sugar and energy stable.

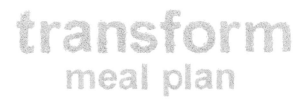

rice: long grain, brown or white

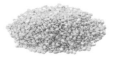

split yellow mung dal

If Your Blood Sugar Crashes

You may need to add more protein to your meals to keep your blood sugar stable. Have a nonfat snack such as an apple and plan to eat more protein at your next meal. See Blood Sugar Balancing on page 36 for more on adding protein. Remember that it can take a few weeks to balance blood sugar, and it's okay if you need to have a snack between meals in the beginning.

*You can bounce back and forth between meal options each day, or even each meal, as needed.

13 Self-Inquiry

Fat metabolism is a great opportunity to face and move through emotional patterns that may have a history of holding you back from greater joy or from realizing your potential. The reason is that molecules of emotion, like some toxins, have been found to store in our fat cells. This includes fat cells in the brain and in other tissues in the body.*

During Phase 2, when fat metabolism really kicks in, I want you to use a journal to document how you feel and what emotional issues and opportunities are arising for you during the cleanse. As you begin to de-stress and these emotions begin to surface, you will likely feel more sensitive and maybe a touch more irritable. These moments of emotional constriction are actually opportunities, if we can recognize them as such, to change our emotional patterns by responding differently than we normally might. To, as I call it, "respond to the *affliction* with *affection*."

Each day during Phase 2, I will give you an exercise to explore in your journal. I call this process "Self-Inquiry," because it gives us the opportunity to look deep within and shake the dust off some patterns and beliefs that may be holding us hostage.

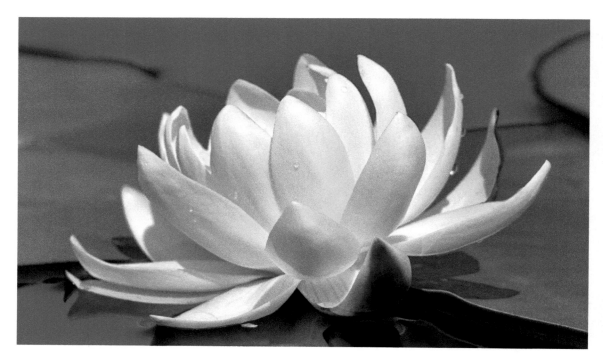

Day 5

What Expands You?

Please list all the things you love:

- List the things that truly expand you. What brings me joy?
- Then ask yourself: am I doing these things?
- If the answer is no, ask: what is keeping me from doing the things I love?
- Now list three qualities you love about your spouse, partner or loved one. Find a way to express your appreciation for these qualities throughout the day.

Day 6

What Contracts You?

Please list all the things that contract you. Opposite to what expands you, these are the things you do not love:

- They can be situations like public speaking, or people like your uncle Fred who is the most selfish, manipulating, intimidating person you know and you never know how to act around him.
- Make a list of people around whom you become a version of you that you don't like.
- List the people around whom you have trouble being your most true, loving self.
- List those people who provoke you and with whom you enter a conversation with your guard up and your weapons ready.
- Pick one of the top offenders on these lists – maybe someone who makes multiple appearances – and write them a love letter, including the things you love or appreciate about them. How did it feel to write that love letter? Write down that feeling as well.

Day 7

Act with Love

Now that you have written a letter of love or appreciation (or two), we are ready for the next step. I realize that writing these letters may have been tough. But if you have surrendered to this process, you may have noticed that letting yourself love them was letting yourself experience the truth of the relationship. Let this letter become the template of truth.

Now, let's take action! Now is the time to use this letter for a model of how you interact with this person. Random acts of love and kindness can be expressed in an email, a note or a quick call of how you really feel. Let yourself express what you wrote in that letter. As you do this you will be breaking old mindsets that have convinced you that you cannot be your wonderful loving self because that person is unsafe, not nice or unworthy of your love. The reality is that when we hold back our true nature, we lose.

Day 8

Drop Childhood Personality Traits

Make a list of personality traits you had to create as a young child to be safe and secure as you were growing up. Who did you have to become?

Then ask yourself, which aspects of that personality are still serving you today and which aspects are not? Which aspects of your personality are holding you back?

Ask yourself: what would I lose if I dropped these personality traits?

Day 9

Take a Risk to Be Joyful and Loving

By now you may be realizing more about your personality traits. You may begin to see that most of what irritates you is a choice. We often try to make others wrong and ourselves right to feel safe. Write down how it feels to be right, and how it feels to make someone wrong. You may notice that being right isn't as great as it seems.

It's time to create more action steps to move through and expose these behavior traits for the illusions they are. If you are afraid of someone or something, create a plan to let yourself be free to interact with them as your open, free and loving self. Make an effort to express affection where you would usually not. It doesn't have to be big, just a subtle way of letting your joy out. Remember, this is your joy and your life. Why should we let anyone keep us from experiencing this most precious part of ourselves?

Take a risk to be joyful and loving!

Day 10

Your Emotional Footprint

Ever wonder what your emotional footprint is like? It is like when you walk through a garden, do the plants expand and reach out to greet you or do they contract and reel out of your way? Do we even know that how we walk through the garden makes an impression on our environment? This is our emotional footprint.

Today, wherever you tread, walk with awareness. Walk with awareness of your own feelings and states, because they project and are palpable to those around us. Walk with awareness of those around you and how your emotional footprint may be impacting them. Play with treading lightly. At the end of the day, take 20 minutes to free-write about how it felt to walk with awareness today.

*Read more about molecules of emotion in my article, "Are Your Emotions Making You Sick?" (lifespa. com/Emotions). Also take the quiz "What's Your Emotional Footprint?" (lifespa.com/EmotionalFoot-print).

Day 11

Day of Rest of Reflection

Use this day to integrate and reflect upon the work you've been doing. Have any new intentions materialized as a result of the Self-Inquiry work? Note them to yourself. Let the power of intention be your greatest ally.

14 Final Flush

Now that we've escorted toxins into the intestinal tract, it's time to flush them out. Laxative therapy, or *virechana* as it's called in Ayurveda, is an important step in this cleanse and a valued therapy in Ayurveda. You can move it a day forward or a day back if you have to, but don't skip it.

Final Flush Protocol

1. The evening of the Final Flush (Day 11), your meal should be very light.

2. Wait 1 – 2 hours after eating supper to take your laxative.

3. Before taking the laxative, take a 15 – 20 minute hot bath to increase circulation to the bowels and relax the abdomen. If a bath is not possible, substitute with a hot shower or rest for 20 minutes with a hot water bottle on your lower abdomen.

4. **Choose the laxative that is best for you:**

   • For sensitive digestion or looser stools, bowel irritation or gallbladder or liver issues: Take 1 ½ cups of prune juice.

   • For normal elimination: Dissolve 1 Tablespoon Epsom salt in 1 cup of water. Add 1 Table-spoon of olive oil and 1 teaspoon of lemon juice.

   • For sluggish, hard or constipated bowels: Dissolve 1 ½ Tablespoon Epsom salt in 1 cup of water. Add 2 Tablespoon of olive oil and 2 teaspoon of lemon juice.

5. You will likely feel a laxative effect in 1 – 15 hours (average time is about 4 – 6 hours).

6. Do not eat anything until the laxative effect has worn off. Sipping room temperature or warm water is ok.

The day after the laxative, you may feel weaker than usual. This is a perfectly common side effect of flushing out your system. The best thing to do is to drink plenty of fluids, staying up on your Hot Sips and Daily Ounces, and to let yourself rest. It will pass!

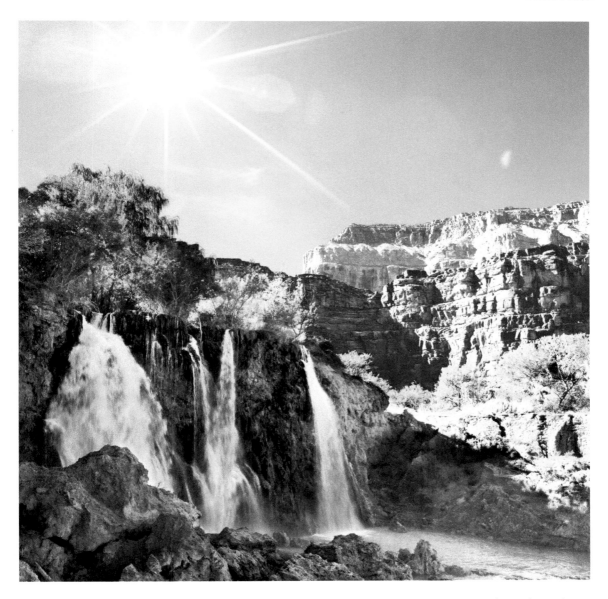

Occasionally, it's possible to not experience a laxative effect. If this happens and you have been eliminating well throughout the cleanse, it's possible your bowels were already flushed out, taking the built-up toxins along. If you haven't been eliminating well, you can take another dose of the laxative therapy the next morning or evening. If you choose to do it in the evening, you can continue with the cleansing diet, but **don't do another day of Morning Ghee.**

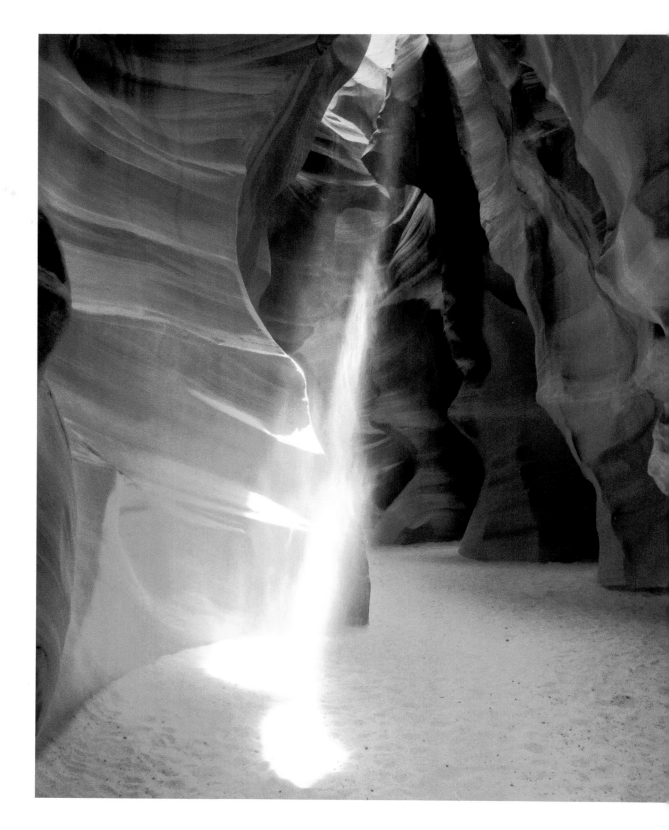

Phase 3
Post-Cleanse

Reset Digestive Strength

15 Reset Digestive Strength

We are going to take these next three days to prepare the body to re-enter into a non-cleansing diet. And while this last phase of the cleanse is likely to involve a pleasant sigh of relief, I also cannot emphasize enough how important it is to do it well.

The object of this phase is twofold: part one is to gently re-enter into the non-cleansing world without shocking the system. Remember, shock or stress will cause the body to store fat rather than to keep burning it. Part two is to finish the job of resetting the digestive strength, which is linked to most chronic health issues.

You'll accomplish this by gradually increasing the herbal formula Beet Cleanse and your digestive formula – Warm or Cool Digest – before each meal for the next three days.* You'll also be drinking lemon water with each meal, letting the acid from the lemon stimulate your digestion, further supporting the work of the herbs.

In Ayurveda, digestive strength is called *agni* – meaning fire. In Ayurvedic thought, the stomach is like a fire that cooks your food, preparing it for assimilation in the small intestine. As we turn the agni back on, you may feel a warm sensation in your belly. This is perfectly normal and a sign that your digestion is reset. At the same time, any actual burning or discomfort is a sign to back off on the herbs.

Digestive Strength Protocol

Here's the Digestive Strength Protocol, which can also be found on pages 18 – 31 of the Day-by-Day Guide.

Day 12:

Take 2 capsules of Beet Cleanse and Warm Digest or Cool Digest,
15 minutes before each meal, with 12 ounces of lemon water.
Sip 4 more ounces of lemon water during the meal.

Day 13:

Take 3 capsules of Beet Cleanse and Warm Digest or Cool Digest,
15 minutes before each meal, with 12 ounces of lemon water.
Sip 4 more ounces of lemon water during the meal.

Day 14:

Take 4 capsules of Beet Cleanse and Warm Digest or Cool Digest,
15 minutes before each meal, with 12 ounces of lemon water.
Sip 4 more ounces of lemon water during the meal.

Note: If you are experiencing any burning or discomfort during the Digestive Strength Protocol,
do not increase the dose of Beet Cleanse and Warm Digest or Cool Digest the following day.

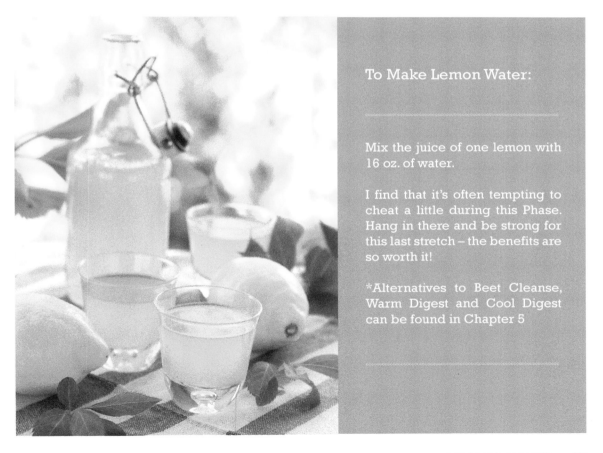

To Make Lemon Water:

Mix the juice of one lemon with 16 oz. of water.

I find that it's often tempting to cheat a little during this Phase. Hang in there and be strong for this last stretch – the benefits are so worth it!

*Alternatives to Beet Cleanse, Warm Digest and Cool Digest can be found in Chapter 5

16 Integration

One of the most common ways of undermining a good cleanse is to binge on hard-to-digest foods, sweets, and stimulants right afterwards. Luckily, Phase 3 takes care of a large chunk of the transition piece, actually priming our digestion so that it can handle foods it may have had trouble with in the past.

Still, putting a little bit of care into how you integrate back into your normal routine is important, and key if you wish to maintain the benefits of fat burning, natural and continual detox, and especially if you are still in the process of finding your healthy balanced weight.

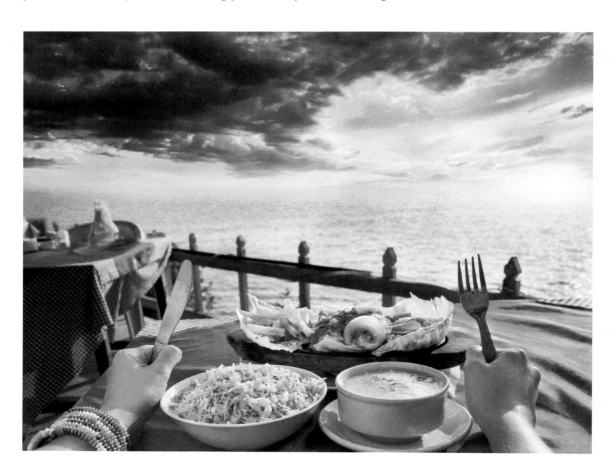

It's quite simple really. Here are the steps:

- Continue the herbal protocol in Chapter 5 until your bottles are empty (you do not need to buy more herbs).

- Continue eating 3 meals a day with no snacks, making the midday meal your largest meal of the day, and having a light and early supper.

- Eat a diet of seasonal foods. Seasonal foods lists for everyday (non-cleansing) life are available on my website at lifespa.com/EatSeasonally *

- If you have lost the desire for heavy foods and wish to continue with a cleansing diet, try eating a diet free of wheat, dairy, and sugar for as long as you are comfortable. This will allow the villi to totally heal and the digestive fire to be fully rekindled.

In Ayurveda, most of the body's wellbeing can be boiled down to proper digestion. By doing the Colorado Cleanse, you're doing an immense service for your digestion and, therefore, every function of your body and mind. You will probably find that you naturally gravitate towards healthier habits in the time following this cleanse. In time, your body will let you know when it needs to cleanse again. Ayurveda recommends cleansing bi-annually in the transitional seasons, once in the fall and once in the spring. The best part is, with each cleanse, your body will become more adept at fat burning, and the cleansing process will become not only easier, but significantly more enjoyable. The benefits are cumulative. It only gets better!

*My book *The 3-Season Diet* goes into depth about eating with the seasons, regularly eating 3 meals a day, and recipe ideas. Find it at lifespa.com/3SeasonDiet

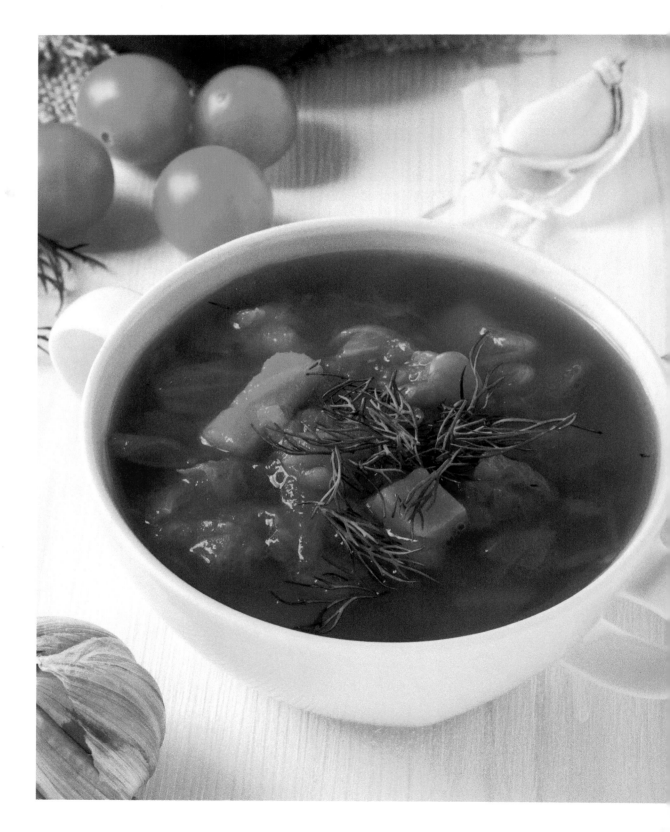

Recipe Inspirations

17 Recipe Inspirations

These recipes are designed to be your launching pad in the kitchen so you can immediately enjoy nourishing and delicious meals that meet the cleansing guidelines.

The recipes are divided into two sections: Spring/Summer and Fall/Winter. Please eat according to the current season for optimal results.

> **Be creative and have fun with your recipes!**
>
> **Make up your own recipes based on the dietary guidelines and**
>
> **Seasonal Cleansing Foods (Appendix 2).**
>
> **Your meals can still be delicious, even while cleansing!**

As this is not a cookbook, we don't go into exact details about how to cook different type of grains, legumes or vegetables. Hopefully you already have this experience or access to another resource about the basics of whole foods cooking. Here are some tips for all phases of the cleanse to support you on your journey:

How to Water Sauté

Instead of sautéing vegetables in oil, water sauté them by bringing a small amount of water to a fast boil in a saucepan, then adding your vegetables and sauté as you would in oil. Add small amounts of water as needed until the vegetables reach their desired consistency.

Puréed Vegetable Soups

You can make vegetable soups by steaming your favorite vegetables and then blending them with vegetable broth or low-fat unsweetened rice milk in a blender. Add lemon, beans (for protein), and seasonal spices. During Phase 1 and 3 you can use seeds for fat and protein. Tip: for ease of digestion, do not add beans and seeds to the same soup – use beans or seeds.

For example:

- *Green Soup: Steamed or raw spinach with cooked split yellow mung dahl beans, garlic, salt, pepper and a dash of lemon juice*
- *Carrot Soup: Steamed carrots with sesame seeds, ginger, turmeric, cumin, salt, pepper*

How to Enjoy Greens

- Many people find greens more palatable when they parboil them for 2-5 minutes in a shallow pan of water, then strain them. This removes the bitter tasting compounds. If you drink the green broth that results, it is surprisingly sweet and buttery!

- Lemon juice helps the greens taste less bitter.

- Collards make a great replacement for tortillas – simply add some rice and beans (or filling of your choice) with sprouts inside a collard leaf and fold like a wrap. You can keep the collard wrap raw or steam it briefly.

- When you steam greens for 8-10 minutes and blend them into a soup with low-sodium vegetable broth, it allows the micronutrients (minerals and vitamins) to become more bio-available.

How Much Salt?

Avoid table salt and enjoy small amounts of healthier alternatives, such as Celtic sea salt, Redmond salt or Himalayan salt.

When we suggest that you add salt in these recipes, we encourage you to use a light hand. Your taste buds will become more sensitive and you will learn to taste the subtle flavors of your food, rather than needing a salty flavor.

How Much Fat?

During Phase 1 and 3, please stick to a low-fat diet. At each meal, choose one source of fat, such as an avocado, 1-2 teaspoons of one type of seed, or 1 Tablespoon of a seed sauce. Do not eat more than one type of fat at a meal to support digestion and fat metabolism.

How to Eat

Enjoy your meal while sitting down, without any distractions such as TV, while working, reading, on the computer, texting, or talking on the phone. Chew your food well and notice the smell and taste of each bite. Sit for a few minutes after you are finished before getting up from the table. Learn more: (lifespa.com/meals).

Fall/Winter Meals for Phase 1 and 3

Breakfast Inspirations
Fall/Winter, Phase 1 and 3

Enjoy some of these breakfast ideas. Be sure to eat enough to carry you through until lunch without triggering a blood sugar crash. You can include a Green Tonic with your morning meal. To enjoy a savory and sustaining breakfast, you can also have any of the Lunch or Dinner Inspirations in the morning.

Sweet Potato Butter with Rice Cakes and Sesame Seeds

- Spread a rice cake with sweet potato butter (purée a sweet potato with a pinch of cinnamon)
- Sprinkle with sesame seeds
- Hot herbal tea (such as cinnamon) or Green Tonic

Bollywood Burrito

- Burrito filled with split yellow mung dahl chili (spice with turmeric, salt, ginger, cumin, cayenne and hing) with onions, corn, and tomatoes. Enjoy wrapped in a raw or steamed collard or kale leaf.
- Rice cakes with avocado, cilantro, lime and salt
- Hot herbal tea (such as ginger) or Green Tonic

Hot Cereal: Basic Whole Oats
Here are two easy ways to cook whole oat groats so they are creamy and easy to digest:

- Crockpot: Rinse 1 cup of whole oats. Add to your crockpot with 4 cups of water and a pinch of salt. Cook on low overnight for 8 hours.
- Stove top: Before bed, soak 1 cup of whole oat groats in a pot with 4 cups of water and a pinch of salt. In the morning, add any additional ingredients. Bring to a boil and cover. Simmer for 1 hour or until oats are soft. Add more water as needed.
- Option: Use rolled oats instead. In a medium saucepan, bring 1/3 cup rolled oats, pinch of salt and 2/3 cup water to a boil. Cover. Reduce heat to low and simmer 5 minutes.
- Flavor with any combo of cinnamon, nutmeg, ginger or cardamom.

Hot Cereal: Ginger Loves Millet

- Add 1 cup of millet to a saucepan with 3 cups of water and 1 grated beet. Add 2 tsp. fresh grated ginger (or 1 tsp. powdered), ½ tsp. cinnamon, ¼ tsp. cloves and ¼ tsp. salt. Bring to a boil. Cover. Simmer 25-30 minutes.
- Top with 1 tsp. flax seeds.
- Hot herbal tea (such as chamomile) or Green Tonic.
- Eat 1 tart apple for dessert.

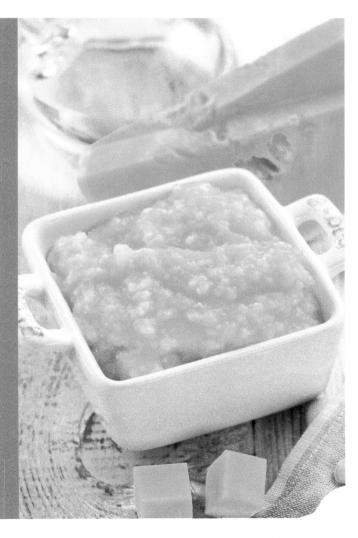

Hot Cereal: 'Pumpkin Pie' Rice Pudding

In a medium saucepan add 1 cup of long grain rice to 2 cups water, 1 cup of cubed sweet potato or winter squash (such as pumpkin), 1 tsp. of cinnamon, 1-2 tsp. fresh grated ginger, ¼ tsp. clove, ¼ tsp. nutmeg and ½ tsp. salt. Bring to a boil. Cover. Reduce heat to low. Simmer about 50 minutes. Remove from heat, let stand, covered, for 5 minutes.

Hot herbal tea (such as clove and orange peel) or Green Tonic.

Eat 1 tart apple for dessert.

Hot Cereal: Kheer Rice Pudding

- Cook 5 cups of rice milk with 1 cup of rice, 2 cinnamon sticks (or 1 tsp. cinnamon), 1 bay leaf, 3 cloves, ¼ tsp. cardamom and ¼ tsp. salt. Bring to a boil. Cover. Reduce heat to low. Simmer until rice is tender (about 20 minutes for white rice, 50 minutes for brown rice).
- Top with 1-2 tsp. hemp seeds and sprinkle with rose water. Chew each bite well to bring out the natural sweetness in the rice.
- Hot herbal tea (Ginger and Cardamom) or Green Tonic.
- Eat 1 tart apple for dessert.

Rosy Pink Amaranth

- In a medium saucepan, add 1 cup of amaranth to 3 cups of water, ½ tsp. of cinnamon, ¼ tsp. salt and add ½ a grated beet. The beet will turn your amaranth a lovely pink color.
- To make it creamy, you can purée it in a blender or food processor, or even with a hand blender.
- For a taste of the exotic and to open the heart, add a splash of rose water.
- Eat 1 tart apple for dessert.

Upma (Traditional South Indian Breakfast)

- Dry roast 1 ½ tsp. cumin seed for 2 minutes. Add ¼" of water, 1/2 cup chopped carrots, 1/2 cup peas, 1 cup of chopped green beans, ½ tsp. of whole black peppercorns and 1 tsp. salt.
- Meanwhile, in a small saucepan, add ½ cup brown rice cereal, 1 ¾ cups of water and a pinch of salt. Bring to a boil while stirring. Reduce heat to low. Cover and simmer for 5 minutes. Remove from heat and stir until smooth.
- Combine the cooked rice cereal with the vegetables and serve.
- Hot herbal tea (such as clove and orange peel) or Green Tonic.
- Eat 1 tart apple for dessert.

Lunch Inspirations
Fall/Winter, Phase 1 and 3

To keep yourself energized and focused until dinner, eat a satisfying lunch between 10am – 2pm when your digestive strength is the strongest.

Colorful Lunch

- Avocado-Tomato Salad with fresh basil and lemon juice
- Root Soup: water sauté 2 sliced celery stalks, 2 diced carrots, 2 chopped parsnips, and 3 chopped beets for a few minutes. Add 1 tsp. salt and enough water to cover vegetables. Cook until tender. Add lemon juice, and salt and pepper.
- Serve with Beet Tonic and/or Green Tonic.
- Eat 1-2 tart apples for dessert.

Pumpkin Soup with Garlic Chard

- Pumpkin soup: water sauté 1 chopped onion and 4-5 cloves of minced garlic until soft. Add 4 cups water, 1 cup puréed canned (or 2 cups cubed fresh) pumpkin, 1 Tbsp. seeded diced jalapeño, 5 diced red potatoes, 1 Tbsp. oregano, pinch of cayenne or other red pepper, and ½ tsp. cumin. Cook until potatoes are soft, about 30 minutes. Add salt and garnish with pumpkin seeds, cilantro or parsley. If you want more protein, add puréed split yellow mung dahl beans as a creamy – and protein rich – base.
- Steam ½ a bunch of chopped chard. Drizzle with 1 Tbsp. Tao of Ginger Dressing (recipe on page 103).
- Serve with rice cakes with avocado and Beet Tonic.
- Eat 1-2 tart apples for dessert.

Sweet Potatoes and Quinoa

- Bake a sweet potato or winter squash in the oven for about 1 hour at 400F. Enjoy plain, or season with salt and pepper or cinnamon.
- Bring 2 ¼ cups of water to a boil with a pinch of salt. Dry roast 1 cup of quinoa in a skillet until it starts to smell nutty. Bring Add quinoa to the boiling water. Add 1 bay leaf, 1 tsp. rosemary and ½ tsp. of sage. Cover. Simmer about 20 minutes, until fluffy.
- Water sauté 1 cup of halved or quartered brussels sprouts in ¼" of water with 1-2 cloves of minced garlic. Drizzle with 1 Tbsp. of Sunny Seed Sauce (recipe on page 102).
- Serve with Beet Tonic and/or Green Tonic.
- Eat 1-2 tart apples for dessert.

Curried Dahl and Aloo Mutter (Potatoes with Peas)

- Split yellow mung bean soup: cook ½ cup of split yellow mung beans with 3 cups of water, 2 chopped tomatoes, 1 tsp. turmeric, ½ tsp. cumin, ½ tsp. ginger powder, ½ tsp. coriander, ¼ tsp. black pepper and a pinch of cayenne. Bring to a boil. Reduce heat to low. Simmer 25-30 minutes, until beans are tender. Add ½ tsp. salt. Garnish with freshly chopped cilantro.
- Aloo Mutter: cover 3 diced potatoes with water and bring to a boil. Add 2 bay leaves. Cook until tender - about 20-25 minutes. Drain and set aside. Meanwhile water sauté 1/2 sliced onion in 1/3 cup water with 1 tsp. coriander, 1 tsp. cumin, ½ tsp. turmeric, ¼ tsp. ground cloves, and ¼ tsp. ginger. Add 1 cup peas and water sauté a few more minutes. Add potatoes. Garnish with lemon juice, salt and pepper.
- Saffron Rice: Add 1 cup of white basmati rice to 1 ¾ cups of boiling water with 1 tsp. salt, pinch of saffron and ½ tsp. turmeric. Bring to a boil. Cover. Reduce heat to low. Simmer 18 minutes. Remove from heat, keep covered and let it stand 5 minutes before serving.
- Serve with Beet Tonic and/or Green Tonic.
- Eat 1-2 tart apples for dessert.

One Pot Lentils and Rice

- In a saucepan, add 1 cup of white basmati rice, 5 cups of water , 1 cup of red lentils, 1 diced parsnip, 1 sliced carrot, 1 stalk of sliced celery, 2 cloves of minced garlic, ½ a chopped onion, ½ tsp. rosemary, ½ tsp. thyme and 2 pinches of salt. Bring to a boil. Cover. Reduce heat to low. Simmer for 20 minutes. Drizzle with 1 Tbsp. of On the Ranch Dressing (recipe in Fall/Winter Side Dishes).
- Serve with Beet Tonic and/or Green Tonic.
- Eat 1-2 tart apples for dessert.

Roots Soup

- Bring 4 cups of water to a boil with a pinch of salt. Dry roast 1 cup of quinoa in a skillet until it starts to smell nutty. Add the quinoa to the boiling water. Add 1-2 cloves of minced garlic, 1 tsp. of fresh grated ginger, 1 diced carrot, 1 sliced turnip, 1 sliced beet and 1 tsp. of salt. Cover. Simmer about 20 minutes, until quinoa and vegetables are tender. Add 1 tsp. sesame seeds. Optional: add 1 tsp. of dulse seaweed flakes.
- Serve with Beet Tonic and/or Green Tonic.
- Eat 1-2 tart apples for dessert.

Mexican Squash Mash with Chili

- Cut a winter squash (such as acorn or butternut) in half, remove seeds, place face down on a baking sheet, add ¼" of water to pan and bake at 400F for 1 hour, or until tender. Mash it with 1 tsp. of your favorite Mexican spice blend (or ½ tsp. cumin, ¼ tsp. chili powder, ½ tsp. paprika, ½ tsp. oregano, ¼ tsp. garlic powder and ¼ tsp. salt).
- Top with fresh corn kernels, thinly sliced red onion, and a few squeezes of lime juice.
- Serve with Lentil Chili: in a saucepan, add 2 cups of water, ½ cup of red lentils with ½ tsp. turmeric, 1-2 tsp. fresh ginger, 1 tsp. cumin, and a pinch of cayenne. Bring to a boil. Cover. Reduce heat to low. Simmer 15 minutes, or until lentils are tender. Garnish with fresh chopped cilantro.
- Serve with Beet Tonic and/or Green Tonic.
- Eat 1-2 tart apples for dessert.

Potato, Leek and Fennel Soup

- Potato soup: water sauté 1 cup of sliced leeks and ½ cup of sliced fresh fennel until soft. Add water and 2 cups diced of potatoes with a pinch of salt and a bay leaf. Simmer until very tender, about 25 minutes. Season with pepper. Garnish with freshly chopped parsley. Serve as is or purée with navy beans or cannellini beans.
- Serve with steamed kale with garlic, salt, pepper and lemon and sunflower seeds.
- Serve with Beet Tonic and/or Green Tonic.
- Eat 1-2 tart apples for dessert.

Corn Chowder

- Water sauté ½ an onion (diced) and 1 garlic clove (minced) until transparent. Add 1-2 stalks of celery (sliced) and sauté for 10 more minutes. Add 1 cup of corn kernels, 2 carrots (sliced in rounds), 1 bay leaf, ½ tsp. salt and 2 cups of water. Simmer for 20 more minutes. Separately blend 1 cup of corn kernels with 4 cups of water, 1 Tbsp. of sunflower seeds, ½ cup of dulse flakes, ¼ tsp. thyme, ¼ tsp. of parsley and ¼ tsp. of pepper. Add to pot and simmer for 10 more minutes. Garnish with fresh parsley.
- Serve with steamed asparagus drizzled with 1 Tbsp. Sunny Seed Sauce (recipe in Fall/Winter Side Dishes). Serve with Beet Tonic and/or Green Tonic.
- Eat 1-2 tart apples for dessert.

Winter Squash Stuffed with Brown Rice

- Cut a winter squash (such as acorn or butternut) in half, remove seeds, place face down on a baking sheet, add ¼" of water to pan and bake at 400F for 1 hour, or until tender.
- Cook the rice: in a saucepan, add 1 cup of brown basmati rice to 2 cups of water and ½ tsp. salt. Bring to a boil. Cover. Reduce heat to low. Simmer for 50 minutes. Remove from heat, keep covered, and let stand for 5 minutes.
- Meanwhile, water sauté in ¼" of water 1 stalk of sliced celery, 2 tsp. of fresh grated ginger, 1 cup of corn, ½ tsp. salt, and ¼ tsp. black pepper.
- Mix the vegetables in with the rice. Spoon into halves of the squash.
- Serve with Beet Tonic and/or Green Tonic.
- Eat 1-2 tart apples for dessert.

Dinner Inspirations
Fall/Winter, Phase 1 and 3

Enjoy an early and light dinner, ideally before 6pm. This will help you digest your dinner more easily and improve the quality of your sleep so you wake up energized and refreshed.

Sun Rays Soup

- Acorn or winter squash soup: cook 2 cups of cubed squash in enough water to cover. Add ½ a chopped onion, 2 cloves of minced garlic, ¼ tsp. salt and ¼ tsp. pepper. You can purée it until creamy if desired. This also tastes delicious with seaweed, such as wakame. Top with sesame seeds.
- Serve with rice cakes with sweet potato butter (see page 94 for recipe).
- Eat 1 tart apple for dessert.

Carrot Soup

- Cook 2 sliced carrots in 1 cup of water with ½ a sliced onion, 1 stalk sliced celery, 1 diced potato, 1 chopped tomato, ¼ tsp. salt and 1 tsp. curry powder. Purée until creamy if desired.
- Serve with a small romaine salad with avocado dressing (lemon, avocado, salt).
- Eat 1 tart apple for dessert.

Borscht

- Cover 2 sliced beets, 1 cup of shredded cabbage and 1 diced onion with 1 ½" of water. Bring to a boil and simmer on low until tender. Mash with a potato masher. Add a dash of lemon juice and salt to taste.
- Serve with rice cakes with a thin layer of avocado.
- Eat 1 tart apple for dessert.

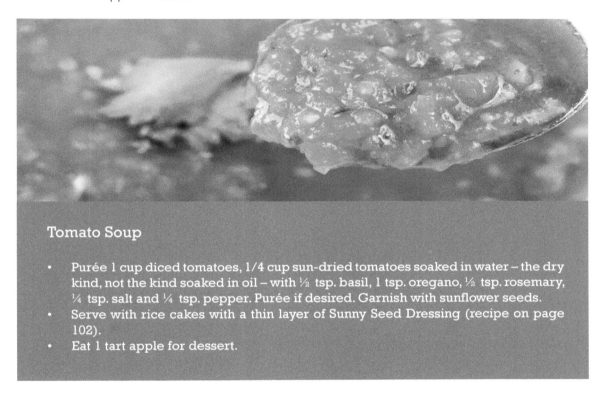

Tomato Soup

- Purée 1 cup diced tomatoes, 1/4 cup sun-dried tomatoes soaked in water – the dry kind, not the kind soaked in oil – with ½ tsp. basil, 1 tsp. oregano, ½ tsp. rosemary, ¼ tsp. salt and ¼ tsp. pepper. Purée if desired. Garnish with sunflower seeds.
- Serve with rice cakes with a thin layer of Sunny Seed Dressing (recipe on page 102).
- Eat 1 tart apple for dessert.

Curried Mung Bean Soup

- In a medium saucepan, add 1 cup of whole green mung beans to 3 cups of water. Add 2 carrots (cut into large chunks), 1 diced potato, 1 sliced onion and 1 tsp. curry powder. Bring to a boil. Cover. Reduce heat to low. Simmer about 1 hour or until beans are tender. Add ¼ tsp. salt after cooking.
- Serve with Turnip-Apple Salad: chop or grate baby turnips and tart apples. Toss with 1 Tbsp. Tao of Ginger Dressing (recipe on page 103).
- Eat 1 tart apple for dessert.

Buckwheat with Savory Vegetables

- In a saucepan, add 1 cup of buckwheat groats to 4-5 cups of water, ½ a diced onion and ½ tsp. salt. Bring to a boil. Reduce heat to low. Cover. Simmer for 30 minutes, or until buckwheat groats are tender.
- Meanwhile, make the gravy: water sauté 1 sliced onion, 1 cup of shredded cabbage, 1 sliced carrot, and 1 tsp. salt until soft.
- Spoon the vegetable gravy on top of the buckwheat. Garnish with 1 tsp. of sesame seeds or 1 Tbsp. Sunny Seed Dressing (recipe at the bottom of this page).
- Eat 1 tart apple for dessert.

Side Dishes and Condiments
Fall/Winter, Phase 1 and 3

Enjoy these side dishes with your lunch or dinner meals. When paired with a Green Tonic and Beet Tonic they could be a completely delicious and nutritious meal.

Condiments for your Rice Cakes

- Cinnamon Sweet Potato Butter: Bake a sweet potato and purée it with a pinch of cinnamon. Tastes like a treat when spread on rice cakes.
- Mexican Bean Pâté: purée 1 cup cooked split yellow mung beans with 1 clove of peeled garlic and 1 tsp. of your favorite Mexican spice blend.
- Tuscan Spread: Purée 1 cup cooked split yellow mung beans with 1 clove of peeled garlic, 1 tsp. rosemary, ¼ tsp. salt and 2 tsp. lemon juice.

Sunny Seed Sauce or Salad Dressing

- Soak ½ a cup of seeds, such as pumpkin seeds, overnight. Rinse. In a blender or food processor, purée the seeds with 1 cup of water, juice of 1/2 lemon, 1 small peeled garlic clove, ½ tsp. salt and ¼ tsp. of pepper.
- Drizzle on vegetables, salads, winter squash or grains.
- If you don't have time to soak the seeds, it is okay – it just may be harder to purée to a creamy consistency if you don't have a high speed blender.
- To keep your meals low-fat, do not add other seeds or avocado to meals that include Sunny Seed Sauce.

On the Ranch Dressing

- Soak ½ a cup of seeds, such as sunflower seeds, overnight. Rinse. In a blender or food processor, purée the seeds with 1 cup of water, juice of 1/2 lemon, 1 small peeled garlic clove, 1 tsp. onion powder, 2 tsp. fresh parsley, ½ tsp. fresh dill chopped (or ¼ tsp. dried), ½ tsp. salt and ¼ tsp. of pepper.
- Please see notes about the Sunny Seed Sauce on the previous page.

The Tao of Ginger Dressing

In a blender or food processor, purée ½ cup of sesame seeds (or tahini) with 1 cup of water, juice of 1/2 lemon, 1-3 small peeled garlic cloves, ½ tsp. salt and ½" – 1" fresh grated ginger.

- Please see notes about the Sunny Seed Sauce on the previous page.

Avocado Dressing

- Mash or purée 1 avocado with the juice of ½ a lemon, ¼ cup water, 1 tsp. fresh dill (or ½ tsp. dried) and ¼ tsp. salt.

Red and White Salad (Turnips and Beets)

- Chop or grate 1 baby turnip with 1 beet. Toss with lemon or one of the dressings above.

Tomato and Corn Salad

- Mix 1 cup of fresh corn kernels with 1 diced tomato, ¼ cup thinly sliced red onion, ¼ cup fresh basil leaves, ¼ tsp. salt and ¼ tsp. black pepper.

Creamy Thai Dressing

- Avocado, lime, cilantro, Serrano, ginger, salt and garlic all puréed with water to desired consistency.

Carrots with Ginger

- Water sauté 2 sliced carrots with 1 tsp. fresh grated ginger in ¼" water. Add water as needed. Add a dash of lemon juice.

Carrots and Turnips

- Cut 2 carrots and 1 turnip into matchstick shapes. Steam until tender. Drizzle with 1 Tbsp. of Tao of Ginger Dressing.

Sliced Turnips with Sweet Potato Butter

- Thickly slice 1 raw turnip. Warm to room temperature. Dip in sweet potato butter.

Garlic Greens

- Water sauté 2 cups of your favorite green vegetable in ¼" water with chopped garlic and ¼ tsp. salt until cooked. Drain off any excess water. Sprinkle with lemon and salt or one of the dressings above.
- Winter Greens: beet greens, mustard greens, kale, chard, collards. You can also use cabbage, brussels sprouts, or broccoli.

Millet with Onions and Carrots

- Layer a saucepan with ½ a diced onion and 2 diced carrots. Add 6 cups of water, 2 cups of millet and ½ tsp. salt. Bring to a boil. Cover. Reduce heat to low. Simmer for 25 minutes, or until millet is tender. Garnish with 1 tsp. of sesame seeds.

Baked Rice

- Preheat oven to 350F. Dry toast 1 cup of long grain brown rice until brown. Place in a baking dish. Pour 3 cups of boiling water over the rice. Cover. Bake 45-50 minutes until the rice is tender and the water is absorbed.
- Option: before cooking, add ½ - 1 cup of seasonal diced vegetables.

Lemon Rice

- In a saucepan, add 1 cup of white basmati rice to 1 ½ cup of water with ½ tsp. salt. Bring to a boil. Cover. Reduce heat to low and simmer for 18 minutes. Remove from heat, keep covered, and let stand for 5 minutes. Add the juice of 2 lemons.

All Fruit Meals
Fall/Winter, Phase 1 and 3

If you wish to eat fruit, Ayurveda recommends that you always eat it separately from other foods. In addition, eat sweet fruits separate from sour fruits and always eat melons separately. Only eat all fruit meals if you have stable blood sugar, and ideally every other day at most. Breakfast is the best time for an all fruit meal.

Zesty Pineapple

- Slice 1 cup of fresh pineapple and garnish with a few pieces of fresh grated ginger and a squeeze of lime.

Sunny Blues (Tangerine Wedges with Blueberries)

- Peel a tangerine and place wedges in a bowl. Garnish with ½ cup of blueberries.

Apple 'Pie'

- Thinly slice 2 tart apples with a mandolin slicer or food processor (or by hand). Toss with lemon juice and 1 tsp. fresh grated ginger and place in an oven safe dish. Sprinkle with ¼ tsp. cardamom and ½ tsp. cinnamon. Bake at 350F for 20-30 for minutes, until apples are soft.

Baked Apples or Pears

- Preheat the oven to 400F. Core your apple and/or pear. Sprinkle the inside of the core with cinnamon and/or nutmeg. Place in a casserole dish and cover. Bake for 30 minutes.

Enchanted Compote

- Place 2 cups of sliced nectarines, apricots and/or peaches into a pot with ¼ cup of water. Add a pinch of clove powder. Bring to a boil. Cover. Reduce heat to low and simmer for 10-15 minutes. Serve warm.

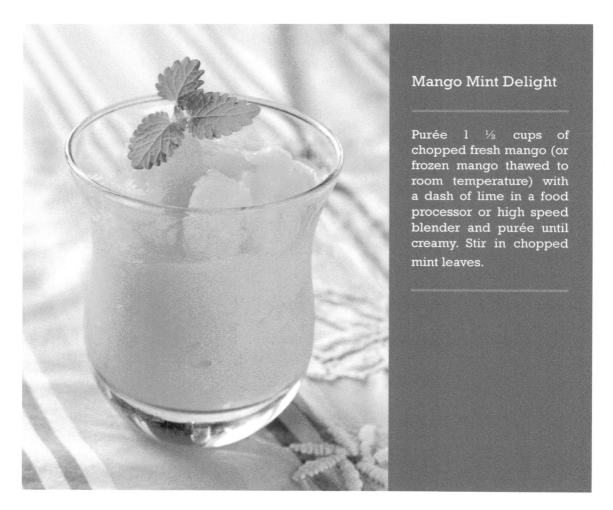

Mango Mint Delight

Purée 1 ½ cups of chopped fresh mango (or frozen mango thawed to room temperature) with a dash of lime in a food processor or high speed blender and purée until creamy. Stir in chopped mint leaves.

Papaya in the Shade of a Palm Tree

- Slice open a ripe papaya. Scoop out the seeds and discard (or make into a salad dressing by puréeing the seeds with avocado, lemon and salt). Sprinkle with lime juice.

Rainbow Fruit Salad – Nature's Skittles

- Toss together ½ cup of blueberries, 6 chopped strawberries, ½ cup chopped pineapple and wedges from 1 tangerine. Sprinkle with lime juice. Marvel at the color. Eat. Enjoy.

Supreme Ojas

- Slice a banana into bite-sized pieces. Garnish with a pinch of cardamom powder and cinnamon.

Spring/Summer Meals for Phase 1 and 3

Breakfast Inspirations
Spring/Summer, Phase 1 and 3

Enjoy some of these breakfast ideas. Be sure to eat enough to carry you through until lunch without getting too hungry or low blood sugar. You can include a Green Tonic with your morning meal. To enjoy a savory and sustaining breakfast, you can also eat any of the Lunch or Dinner inspirations in the morning.

Avocado and Rice Cakes

- Spread avocado and a dash of salt on your favorite rice cake. Add 1 tsp. of seeds, such as sunflower, for protein. Surprisingly satisfying!
- Eat 1 tart apple for dessert.

Hot Cereal: Rice Cream Dream

- In a saucepan, add ½ cup of long grain rice to 2 cups of water with ½ tsp. salt, ½ tsp. cinnamon and ¼ cardamom. Bring to a boil. Cover. Simmer for 50 minutes. Remove from heat, keep covered and let it stand for 5 minutes before serving. (Fast track: use brown rice cereal and follow the instructions on the package. It usually takes 5-8 minutes to cook).
- Option: purée in a blender or food processor with ¼ cup of rice milk.
- Garnish with 1 tsp. flax seeds.
- Eat 1 tart apple for dessert.

Hot Cereal: Basic Whole Oats
Here are two easy ways to cook whole oat groats so they are creamy and easy to digest:

- Crockpot: Rinse 1 cup of whole oats. Add to your Crockpot with 4 cups of water and a pinch of salt. Cook on low overnight for 8 hours.

- Stove top: Before bed, soak 1 cup of whole oat groats in a pot with 4 cups of water and a pinch of salt. In the morning, add any additional ingredients. Bring to a boil and cover. Simmer for 1 hour or until oats are soft. Add more water as needed.
- Option: Use rolled oats instead. In a medium saucepan, bring 1/3 cup rolled oats, pinch of salt and 2/3 cup water to a boil. Cover. Reduce heat to low and simmer 5 minutes.
- Eat 1 tart apple for dessert.

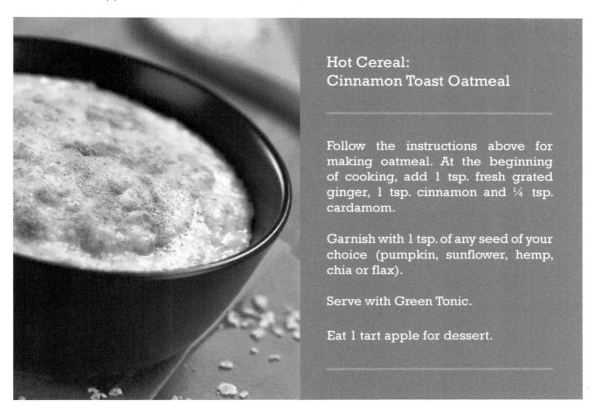

Hot Cereal: Cinnamon Toast Oatmeal

Follow the instructions above for making oatmeal. At the beginning of cooking, add 1 tsp. fresh grated ginger, 1 tsp. cinnamon and ¼ tsp. cardamom.

Garnish with 1 tsp. of any seed of your choice (pumpkin, sunflower, hemp, chia or flax).

Serve with Green Tonic.

Eat 1 tart apple for dessert.

Millet with Chives

- Toast 1/2 cup of millet in a medium saucepan at medium heat for 3-5 minutes. Add 1 ½ cups of water, 1 minced garlic clove and ¼ tsp. salt. Bring to a boil. Cover. Reduce heat to low. Simmer 25 minutes, or until cooked.
- Garnish with chopped chives and 1 tsp. sesame seeds.
- Serve with Green Tonic.
- Eat 1 tart apple for dessert.

Lunch Inspirations
Spring/Summer, Phase 1 and 3

To keep yourself energized and focused until dinner, eat a satisfying lunch between 10am – 2pm when your digestive strength is the strongest. Do not eat with any distractions such as TV, while working, reading, on the computer, or talking on the phone. Sit for a few minutes after you are finished before getting up from the table. Learn more: (lifespa.com/meals).

Buddha Bowl: Veggies, Grains and Beans

Rice and Beans: Cook your favorite grain with your favorite beans and spices. Choose from these grains: amaranth, buckwheat, millet, quinoa, brown or white long grain rice. Then choose from these legumes: adzuki, garbanzo, fava, kidney, lentils, lima, mung and split pea. Here are some ideas:

- Adzuki beans with millet, garlic, and ginger
- Lentils with quinoa and curry
- Garbanzo beans with white long grain rice, Italian herbs and garlic
- Kidney beans and brown basmati rice with (mild) Mexican or Cajun spices
- Enjoy with a salad or steamed vegetables from the Spring Cleansing Grocery List. Drizzle with 1 Tbsp. of one of the sauces or dressings in Spring/Summer Side Dishes.
- Serve with Beet Tonic and/or Green Tonic.
- Eat 1-2 tart apples for dessert.

Vegetable Soup, Beans/Chicken and Kale
From *The 3-Season Diet* by John Douillard

- Vegetable Soup (made with cooked rice or quinoa, carrots, green beans, celery, dandelions, mushrooms and onions mixed in blender)
- Rice cake with avocado and salt
- Steamed kale (with lemon, salt, black pepper and garlic)
- Vegetarian option: baked beans (with basmati rice and asparagus)
- Non-Vegetarian option (only if needed to stabilize blood sugar): Grilled chicken breast (skinless and boneless, marinated in ginger-tamari sauce and grilled)
- Serve with Beet Tonic and/or Green Tonic.
- Eat 1-2 tart apples for dessert.

Greens and More Greens
From *The 3-Season Diet* by John Douillard

- Mixed Green Salad (with papaya slices, lime, a pinch of salt)
- Sautéed mixed greens (made with dandelions, spinach and mustard greens, water-sautéed with garlic and onions)
- Vegetarian option: Garbanzo bean casserole (made with rice, carrots, onions, fresh corn, tomato sauce, cayenne, coriander and sage)
- Serve with Beet Tonic and/or Green Tonic.
- Eat 1-2 tart apples for dessert.

Spinach Salad and Artichokes
From *The 3-Season Diet* by John Douillard

- Spinach Salad (made with sliced mushrooms and tossed with lemon and salt)
- Steamed Artichoke (with oregano, basil, bay leaf, and marjoram)
- Mixed Green Vegetables (steamed green beans, cabbage, and broccoli with marjoram and puréed turnips and carrots)
- Vegetarian option: Indian Style Rice and Beans (long-grain brown rice and split mung beans with turmeric, ginger and black pepper)
- Serve with Beet Tonic and/or Green Tonic.
- Eat 1-2 tart apples for dessert.

Herbed Rice with Green Beans

- Add 1 cup white basmati rice to 1 ½ cups of water in a pot. Add 1-2 cloves of minced garlic, ½ cup of chopped shallots or onion, ½ cup chopped asparagus, ¼ tsp. chili flakes and ½ tsp. salt. Bring to a boil. Cover. Simmer 18 minutes. Remove from heat, keep covered, and let it stand for 5 minutes before garnishing with salt, pepper and fresh basil leaves.
- Green Bean Salad: Water sauté 1 cup of chopped green beans with 2 tsp. minced garlic, ½ tsp. thyme, ¼ tsp. chili powder, ¼ tsp. salt and ¼ tsp. black pepper. Garnish with fresh bell pepper and some minced red onion).
- Spinach Salad with 1 Tbsp. DaffoDILL Dressing (recipe on page 116).
- Serve with Beet Tonic and/or Green Tonic.
- Eat 1-2 tart apples for dessert.

Black Bean Soup

- Soak 2 cups of black beans overnight. Rinse. Place in a pot with 4 cups of water. Bring to a boil. Cover. Reduce heat to low and simmer for 1 hour. Add ½ chopped onion, 2 cloves of minced garlic, 1 tsp. coriander, 1 ½ tsp. cumin and 1 pinch of cayenne. Cook until tender. Finish with ½ tsp. salt and juice of ½ a lemon.
- Enjoy with a rice cake with avocado and salt.
- Serve with Beet Tonic and/or Green Tonic.
- Eat 1-2 tart apples for dessert.

Red Beans and Rice

- Cook kidney beans (or use 2 cups of canned kidney beans): soak 2 cups of kidney beans overnight. Rinse. Add to a pot with 6 cups of water. Bring to a boil for 10 minutes, then cover and reduce heat to low. Simmer for 1 ½ hours or until beans are tender. Crockpot method: place the soaked and rinsed kidney beans into a crockpot with 6 cups of water and cook on low for 8-10 hours.
- Water sauté 1 stalk of sliced celery and 1 cup of diced red bell pepper for 10 minutes. Add 1 tsp. thyme, 1 tsp. oregano, 1 tsp. paprika, 1 tsp. pepper and ½ tsp. salt. Add this mixture to the cooked beans.
- Serve the beans on top of the rice.
- Serve with Beet Tonic and/or Green Tonic.
- Eat 1-2 tart apples for dessert.

Dinner Inspirations
Spring/Summer, Phase 1 and 3

Enjoy an early and light dinner, ideally before 6pm. This will help you digest your dinner more easily and improve the quality of your sleep. You will also wake up more energized.

Split Pea Soup
From *The 3-Season Diet* by John Douillard

- Split Pea Soup (made with rice and carrots, celery, onions and garlic)
- Rice cake with avocado and salt
- Eat 1 tart apple for dessert.

Cream of Spinach Soup
From *The 3-Season Diet* by John Douillard

- Cream of Spinach Soup (made with rice milk, ginger, paprika, black pepper, and cooked spinach, blended and cooled)
- Rice cake with avocado and salt
- Eat 1 tart apple for dessert.

Chickpea Soup
From *The 3-Season Diet* by John Douillard

- Garbanzo Soup (made with puréed garbanzo beans and chopped asparagus, cumin, cayenne, garlic and coriander, then garnished with fresh cilantro and lemon)
- Chopped asparagus with fresh parsley and a squeeze of lemon
- Serve with rice cakes
- Eat 1 tart apple for dessert.

Szechuan Not-Fried Rice

- Szechuan Fried Rice: Cook ½ cup of long grain brown rice in 1 cup of water with ¼ tsp. salt. Bring to a boil. Cover. Reduce heat to low. Simmer for 50 minutes. Remove from heat, keep covered and let stand for 5 minutes. Meanwhile, water sauté 1 tsp. fresh ginger, 2 cloves of minced garlic, ¼ tsp. red chili pepper, ½ cup shiitake mushroom and 1 diced red bell pepper for 10 minutes. Add ½ cup of peas and 1 cup of spinach. Cook for 5 more minutes. Add 1 cup of cooked adzuki beans and toss with rice. Garnish with 1 tsp. sesame seeds.
- Serve with Beet Tonic (with ginger).
- Eat 1 tart apple for dessert.

Nourishing Rice Salad

- First, cook the rice: in a saucepan, add 1 cup of long grain brown rice to 2 cups of water and ½ tsp. salt. Bring to a boil. Cover. Reduce heat to low and simmer for 50 minutes. Remove from heat, keep covered and let stand for 5 minutes.
- Toss with 1 chopped green onion, 2 Tbsp. fresh chopped parsley, 1 cup of cooked peas, 2 Tbsp. lemon juice, 1 tsp. salt and 1 Tbsp. pine nuts or one of the dressings in the Spring/ Summer Side Dishes.
- Eat 1 tart apple for dessert.

Green and White Soup

- Bring 5 cups of water to a boil. Add 4 cups of diced parsnips. Bring back to a boil. Simmer for 15 minutes. Purée in a food processor or high speed blender. Return to the pot and add 1 cup of broccoli florets. Simmer for 15-20 more minutes. Season with salt and pepper to taste. Garnish with pine nuts.
- Eat 1 tart apple for dessert.

Zen Spring Soup

- Bring 4 cups of water to a boil with a pinch of salt. Dry roast 1 cup of quinoa in a skillet until it starts to smell nutty. Add quinoa to the boiling water. Add 1-2 cloves of minced garlic, 1 tsp. of fresh grated ginger, 1 cup of shredded cabbage, 1 sliced carrot, and 1 diced turnip. Cover. Simmer about 20 minutes, until quinoa and vegetables are tender. Add 1 tsp. of salt. Optional: add 1 tsp. of dulse seaweed flakes.
- Steam 1 cup of bok choy. Drizzle with 1 Tbsp. of Tao of Ginger Sauce (recipe in Fall/Winter Side Dishes).
- Eat 1 tart apple for dessert.

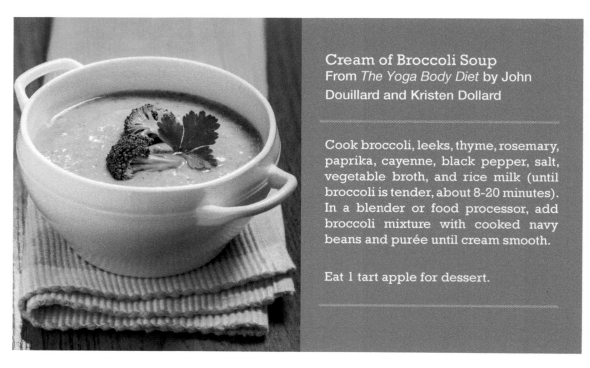

Cream of Broccoli Soup
From *The Yoga Body Diet* by John Douillard and Kristen Dollard

Cook broccoli, leeks, thyme, rosemary, paprika, cayenne, black pepper, salt, vegetable broth, and rice milk (until broccoli is tender, about 8-20 minutes). In a blender or food processor, add broccoli mixture with cooked navy beans and purée until cream smooth.

Eat 1 tart apple for dessert.

Personal Pizza
From *The Yoga Body Diet* by John Douillard and Kristen Dollard

- Spread 2 slices of rice cakes with tomato paste. Top with minced garlic, bell pepper, spinach and pineapple slices. Bake for 5 minutes. Sprinkle with salt and basil.
- Eat 1 tart apple for dessert.

Quinoa Tabouli

- Cook the quinoa: Bring 2 ¼ cups of water to a boil with a pinch of salt. Dry roast 1 cup of quinoa in a skillet until it starts to smell nutty. Add quinoa to the boiling water. Add ½ tsp. of salt. Cover. Simmer about 20 minutes, until fluffy.
- Toss with ½ cup of peas, ½ diced cucumber, 2-3 Tbsp. minced chives, 2 Tbsp. fresh chopped parsley, ½ tsp. thyme, ½ tsp. marjoram, 3 Tbsp. lemon juice, ½ tsp. salt and ¼ tsp. black pepper.
- Serve with Green Tonic and/or Beet Tonic.
- Eat 1 tart apple for dessert.

Side Dishes and Condiments
Spring/Summer, Phase 1 and 3

Tuscany Dressing

- Soak ½ a cup of seeds, such as sunflower seeds, overnight. Rinse. In a blender or food processor, purée the seeds with 1 cup of water, juice of 1/2 lemon, 1 small peeled garlic clove, ½ tsp. basil, ½ tsp. oregano, ½ tsp. salt and ¼ tsp. of pepper.
- Drizzle on vegetables, salads, winter squash or grains.
- If you don't have time to soak the seeds, it is okay – it just may be harder to purée to a creamy consistency if you don't have a high speed blender.
- To keep your meals low-fat, do not add other seeds or avocado to meals that include Tuscany Dressing.

Minty Tahini Sauce

- In a blender or food processor, purée ½ cup of sesame seeds (or tahini) with 1 cup of water, ½ tsp. salt, 1-2 cloves of peeled garlic, juice of 1 lemon and 1 bunch of fresh mint leaves.
- Variation: omit the mint to make Lemon Tahini Sauce.
- See notes about Tuscany Dressing on the previous page.

DaffoDILL Dressing

- In a blender or food processor, purée ½ cup of pine nuts (or other seed) with 1 cup of water, juice of 1/2 lemon, 1 small peeled garlic clove, 1 bunch of fresh dill (or 1 tsp. dried) and ½ tsp. salt.
- Please see notes about Tuscany Dressing on the previous page.

Avo Pesto

- Mash or blend ½ cup of chopped avocado, ¼ cup of chopped fresh herbs (such as basil, cilantro, parsley or arugula), with juice of ½ a lemon and ¼ tsp. of salt.
- Spread on grains, rice cakes, or romaine 'boats' (whole leaves).
- Add ¼ cup of water to make it a sauce or dressing.

Condiments for your Rice Cakes

- Cinnamon Sweet Potato Butter: Bake a sweet potato and purée it with a pinch of cinnamon. Tastes delicious spread on rice cakes.
- Apple butter
- Mexican Bean Pâté: purée 1 cup cooked split yellow mung beans with 1 clove of peeled garlic and 1 tsp. of your favorite Mexican spice blend.
- Avo Pesto – recipe above.

Emerald Apple Sauce

- In a food processor (or by hand), grate 2 tart apples, 1-2 tsp. fresh ginger, ½ tsp. cinnamon and a handful of chopped fresh parsley. The parsley tastes surprisingly divine. Start with a small amount if you aren't sure. You can even go up to a whole cup – or more!
- Lasts up to 2 days in the fridge.

Cool as a Carrot Salad

- In a food processor (or by hand), grate 3 carrots and 1 beet. Toss with lemon juice and 1 tsp. of sunflower seeds or Minty Tahini Sauce.

Sunset Cauliflower and Carrots

- Steam 1-2 sliced carrots and 1 cup of cauliflower florets. Drizzle with Minty Tahini Sauce.

Millet Mashed Potatoes

- Lightly roast 2 cups of millet in a skillet, until it smells nutty.
- In a separate sauce pan, bring 7 cups of water to a boil. Add the millet to the water, along with 2 cups of chopped cauliflower and ¼ tsp. salt. Bring to a boil. Cover. Reduce heat to low and simmer for 25 minutes. Purée until smooth in a food processor or high speed blender, and add water as needed. Top with chives.

Arugula Salad

- Toss 2 cups of arugula with 1 serving of Avo Pesto. Add ½ a grated beet.

Happy Sprouts Salad

- Drizzle 1 cup of sprouts (such as sunflower, pea, alfalfa or radish) with 1 Tbsp. of dressing, such as the Tuscany Dressing (recipe on page 15).

Cucumber 'Chips'

- Thickly slice one crisp cucumber. Garnish lightly with 1 tsp. of roasted sesame seeds and ¼ tsp. of salt.

Mediterranean Spinach

- Steam spinach in a steamer basket for 4-5 minutes. Garnish with a pinch of salt, nutmeg, cinnamon and a squeeze of lemon.

All Fruit Meals
Spring/Summer, Phase 1 and 3

If you wish to eat fruit, Ayurveda recommends that you always eat it separately from other foods. In addition, eat sweet fruits separate from sour fruits and always eat melons separately. Only eat all fruit meals if you have stable blood sugar, and ideally every other day at most. Breakfast is the best time for an all fruit meal.

Summer in a Bowl

- Toss 6 sliced strawberries with 1 cup of chopped oranges.
- Optional: add a handful of pomegranate seeds.
- Garnish with fresh mint leaves.

Papaya with Lime and Chili

- Halve a papaya and remove the seeds (you can actually eat a few spoonfuls of the pungent seeds as they are excellent for your digestion). Sprinkle with lime juice and a dash of chili powder.

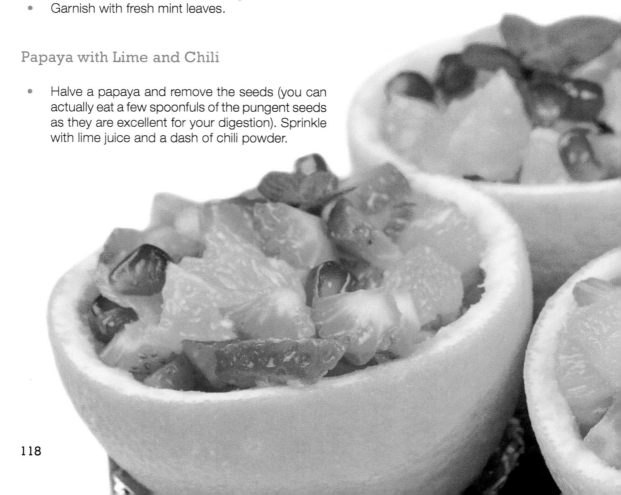

Pears with Peach 'Fondue'

- Purée 1 fresh peach in a blender or food processor. Add a little water if needed.
- Dip 1 sliced pear into this sauce for an easy "fondue."

Apples with Cinnamon

- Slice 1-2 tart apples and toss with a dash of lemon juice and sprinkle with ¼ tsp. cinnamon and a pinch of nutmeg.

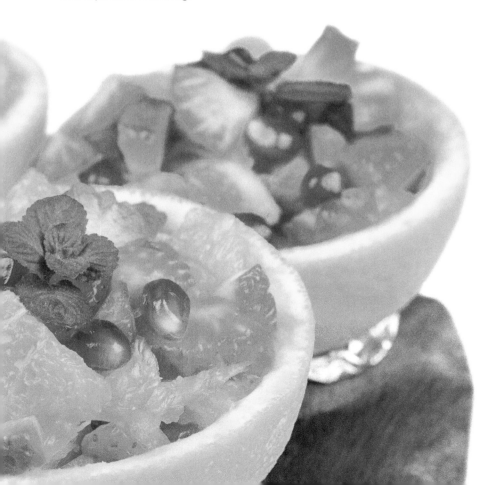

Recipes and Meals for Phase 2

Feel free to be creative with your own during Phase 2. Just keep in mind these main guidelines:

- Keep it NONfat.
- Use vegetables from the Seasonal Cleansing Foods in Appendix 2. Eat more cooked vegetables than raw.
- Follow the Meal Options in Chapter 12.
- If you are following the Rejuvenate or Nourish meal options, you can use any of the recipes for Phase 1 and 3 without the fat (no seeds or avocado). Choose from the Fall/Winter or Spring/Summer recipes based on the current season.
- Though white basmati rice and split yellow mung dahl beans are the most detoxifying, you can use your favorite whole grain and legumes (such as quinoa and lentils or millet and adzuki beans).
- Ensure that your meals are warm and moist or brothy (such as stews or soups).
- Use spices such as ginger, cumin, turmeric, black pepper and coriander to aid with digestion. Avoid spicy foods or flavors as our goal is to heal the intestinal villi.

Look for the symbol next to each recipe that matches which meal plan you are following:

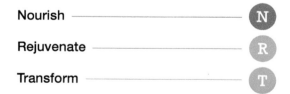

Kitchari Recipe

The recipe below makes enough for 3-4 meals. You can adjust the spices to your taste (m. people like to double or triple the spices).

1   cup Split Yellow Mung Dahl Beans* (see 'weak digestion' below)
1   cup white basmati rice
1   Tbsp. fresh ginger root (add more if you like ginger)
½   tsp. turmeric powder
½   tsp. coriander powder
½   tsp. cumin powder
½   tsp. whole cumin seeds
½   tsp. brown or yellow mustard seeds
1   pinch hing (also called asafetida or asafoetida) optional
8   cups of water or vegetable broth
½   tsp. salt (rock salt is best). You can add more if you wish.
1   small handful fresh chopped cilantro leaves

- Wash split yellow mung beans (dahl) and rice together until water runs clear.
- Heat a large pot on medium heat and then add ginger root, turmeric, coriander powder, cumin powder, whole cumin seeds, mustard seeds, and hing. This dry-roasting will enhance the flavor. Stir all together for a few minutes. Be careful to avoid burning.
- Add dahl and rice and stir again so all the grains and beans are covered with the spices.
- Add water and bring to a boil. Boil for 10 minutes.
- Turn heat to low, cover pot and cook until dahl and rice become soft (about 30-40 min).
- The cilantro leaves and salt can be added just before serving.

More About Split Yellow Mung Dahl beans:

It's important to use split yellow mung dahl beans as they are easy to digest because the hard to digest husk falls off when split. Split yellow mung dahl beans have cleansing qualities that pull toxins from the body. They are available at Asian or Indian grocery stores (be careful of yellow dye) or through LifeSpa. Different spellings include "moong" and/or "dal". Do not use whole mung dahl beans, which are green, or yellow split peas or lentils.

For Weak Digestion, Gas or Bloating

- Before starting to prepare the kitchari, soak the split yellow mung dahl beans overnight. Drain and rinse before cooking.
- Or, parboil the beans by covering with water and bringing to a boil. Drain and rinse. Repeat 2-3 times:

Rice Cooker Method

Nice and Easy! Follow the guidelines above for soaking or parboiling the beans. Dry roast the spices for best taste, then throw everything into your rice cooker for effortless kitchari! You can take your rice cooker to work and even travel!

Flavor Options

Instead of using the spices in the recipe above, you can play around with your favorite blend of seasonings. It is best to stay away from anything spicy, such as Mexican, Southwest, Thai, Caribbean, or Cajun flavors.

Here are some ideas:

1	**Breakfast: make it delicious with cinnamon, ginger, nutmeg and a splash of nonfat rice milk.**	N R T
2	**Simple: salt and a squeeze of lemon juice.**	N R T
3	**'Pasta' Kitchari: Make it plain with garlic powder, salt, and pepper.**	N R T
4	**Refreshing Kitchari: salt, with fresh dill, cilantro and a squeeze of lemon.**	N R
5	**Italian: add Italian seasoning and 2-5 Tbsp. of tomato paste.**	N R
6	**Cauliflower Kitchari: add roasted cauliflower and nonfat salsa.**	N R
7	**Prunes: cook prunes into the kitchari with a few cloves (only if you are experiencing constipation).**	N R

Breakfast Inspirations – Phase 2

Be sure to eat enough breakfast to carry you through until lunch without getting too hungry or having low blood sugar. You can cook kitchari or hot cereals in a crockpot overnight so that you wake up to a warm breakfast. During Phase 2, if you are following the Nourish meal option, you can use any of the recipes for Phase 1 and 3 – just remove any avocado or seeds.

Rice Milk

- You can make this rice milk to drink with your morning ghee or as a splash of milk for your hot cereal.
- Add 1/3 cup of brown rice to 1 cup of boiling water. Bring to a boil again. Cover, reduce heat to low and summer 40-50 minutes, until rice is cooked. Place the rice in a blender and add 3 cups of warm water. Blend until smooth, about 2 minutes. Add more water to reach your desired consistency. You can strain it if you like with a piece of cheesecloth, nut milk bag or fine mesh strainer.

Hot Cereal: Cinnamon Kitchari

- Follow the kitchari recipe, but use ½ – 1 tsp. of cinnamon instead of the other spices. You can also add ginger and/or cardamom.
- To make it creamy, you can purée it in a blender or food processor, or even with a hand blender.
- If you add hot water, you can make it thin enough to drink like a 'smoothie' for a new texture experience.
- Hot herbal tea (such as chamomile).

Hot Cereal: Brown Rice with Ginger and Cardamom

- In a medium saucepan, add ½ cup long grain brown rice, 1 cup of water, 1 tsp. fresh grated ginger, ¼ tsp. salt and a pinch of cardamom. Bring to a boil. Cover. Reduce heat to low. Simmer for 50 minutes. Remove from heat, keep covered, and let stand for 5 minutes before serving.
- To make it creamy, you can purée it in a blender or food processor, or even with a hand blender.
- Hot herbal tea (such as dandelion root).

Hot Cereal: Creamy Kitchari with Cinnamon

- Follow the kitchari recipe, but use ½ tsp. – 1 tsp. of cinnamon instead of the other spices. You can also add ginger and/or cardamom.
- To make it creamy, you can purée it in a blender or food processor, or even with a hand blender.
- If you add hot water, you can make it thin enough to drink like a 'smoothie' for a new texture experience.
- Hot herbal tea (such as chamomile).

Rosy Pink Kitchari

- Follow the kitchari recipe, but cook it plain with ½ tsp. – 1 tsp. of cinnamon, instead of the spices, and add ½ a beet (peeled and chopped). The beet will turn your kitchari a lovely pink color.
- To make it creamy, you can purée it in a blender or food processor, or even with a hand blender.
- For a taste of the exotic and to open the heart, add a splash of rose water.
- Hot herbal tea (such as ginger and orange peel).

Hot Cereal: Savory Millet with Greens

- Dry-roast ½ cup of millet in a sauce pan on medium high until it tastes nutty – about 3-5 minutes. Add to a pot with 1 ½ cups of water, ½ tsp. salt and 1 tsp. fresh grated ginger. Bring to a boil. Cover. Reduce heat to low. Simmer for 25 minutes, or until millet is tender.
- Meanwhile, water sauté or steam 2 cups of seasonal vegetables.
- Serve the millet in a bowl with the greens on top.
- Sprinkle with seaweed, such as dulse flakes.
- Hot herbal tea (such as a mix of orange peel, cinnamon and clove).

Lunch and Dinner Inspirations – Phase 2

Lunch Tips

To keep yourself energized and focused until dinner, eat a satisfying lunch between 10am – 2pm when your digestive strength is strongest. Do not eat with any distractions, such as TV, working, reading, computer, texting, or talking on the phone. Sit for a few minutes after you are finished before getting up from the table.

Dinner Tips

Enjoy an early and light dinner, ideally before 6pm. This will help you digest your dinner more easily and improve the quality of your sleep so you wake up more energized.

Kitchari

- If you like, you can eat this for every meal during the Colorado Cleanse.
- Follow the kitchari recipe and any of the flavor options for variety.
- Take a deep breath and smell your kitchari while noticing the color and texture with your eyes.
- Chew each bite mindfully.

Herbed Rice and Italian Dahl

- Herbed Rice: Cook 1 cup of white basmati rice in 1 ½ cups of low sodium vegetable broth with 2-3 cloves of minced garlic. Garnish with salt, pepper and ¼ cup of fresh basil leaves (minced). If you don't have fresh basil leaves, you can cook 2 tsp. of dried basil leaves into the rice.
- Italian Dahl: cook 1 cup of split yellow mung dahl beans in 2 cups of water with 1 tsp. rosemary, 1 tsp. oregano, 2 cloves of minced garlic and lemon juice, salt and pepper to taste.
- Nourish and Rejuvenate meal plan: you can serve with steamed seasonal vegetables drizzles with lemon juice, sea salt and pepper to taste.

Flavor-Full Dahl and Saffron Rice

- Flavor-Full Dahl: Dry roast for a few minutes: 2 whole cloves, 1 tsp. cumin seeds, ½ tsp. mustard seeds and 8 fenugreek seeds. Add 1/8 tsp. ginger powder and ½ tsp. cardamom. Cook for 1 more minute. Add 4 cups of water and 1 cup of split yellow mung dahl beans. Bring to a boil. Cover. Reduce heat to low and simmer until creamy, about 30 minutes. Add sea salt to taste.
- Saffron Rice: in a saucepan, add 1 cup of white basmati rice to 1 ½ cups of water with ½ tsp. salt, 8-10 threads of saffron and 1 tsp. of mustard seeds. Bring to a boil. Cover. Reduce heat to low. Simmer for 18 minutes. Remove from heat, keep covered and let it stand for 5 minutes.
- To serve, spoon the curried dahl over the saffron rice.
- Nourish and Rejuvenate meal plan: you can serve with steamed seasonal vegetables drizzled with lemon juice, sea salt and pepper to taste.

Soothing Dahl with Winter Greens

- Soothing Dahl: in a saucepan, add 2 cups split yellow mung bean soup in 4 cups water with 2 tsp. turmeric, 1 tsp. cumin, 1 tsp. ginger powder (or 2 tsp. fresh grated), 1 tsp. coriander, and a pinch of hing (also called asafoetida). Bring to a boil. Cover. Reduce heat to low. Simmer for 20 minutes. Add 2-3 cups of your favorite chopped seasonal vegetables. Add ½ tsp. salt and ¼ tsp. black pepper.
- Serve with Yellow Rice: In a saucepan, add 1 cup of white basmati rice to 1 ½ cups of water with ½ tsp. salt and 1 tsp. turmeric. Bring to a boil. Cover. Reduce heat to low. Simmer for 18 minutes. Remove from heat, keep covered and let it stand for 5 minutes.
- Nourish and Rejuvenate meal plan: you can serve with steamed seasonal vegetables drizzles with lemon juice, sea salt and pepper to taste.

Italian Lentil Soup with Rosemary-Garlic Rice

- To make the soup: cook 1 cup of green lentils (or any lentil) in 3 cups of water with ½ tsp. each of oregano, basil, rosemary, thyme and sage. Bring to a boil. Cover. Reduce heat to low and simmer until the lentils are tender, about 25-30 minutes. Garnish with ¼ cup fresh parsley (chopped), and sea salt and black pepper to taste.
- To make the Rosemary-Garlic Rice: in a saucepan, add 1 cup of long grain brown rice and 2 cups of water with 2 tsp. rosemary, 2-3 cloves of minced garlic and sea salt.
- Nourish and Rejuvenate meal plan: you can serve with steamed seasonal vegetables drizzles with lemon juice, sea salt and pepper to taste.

Moroccan Lentil Stew with Beet Greens

- Cook 1 cup of red lentils (or any small bean) in 3 cups water with the following spices: 1 tsp. cinnamon, 1 tsp. cumin, ½ tsp. ginger powder (or 1 tsp. fresh grated), ¼ tsp. cloves, ¼ tsp. nutmeg, ¼ tsp. turmeric and 1/8 tsp. curry powder. Bring to a boil. Cover. Reduce heat to low and simmer until lentils are soft, about 20 minutes. Add ½ tsp. salt.
- Brown rice: in a saucepan, add 1 cup of long grain brown rice, 2 cups of water and ½ tsp. salt. Bring to a boil. Cover. Reduce heat to low. Simmer for 50 minutes. Remove from heat, keep covered and let stand for 5 minutes before serving.
- Meanwhile, water sauté chopped greens. Garnish with a squeeze of lemon and a dash of salt.
- Nourish and Rejuvenate meal plan: you can add 2 cups of chopped seasonal vegetables at the very beginning of cooking the stew.

Vegetable Soup

- Chop 2-4 cups of seasonal vegetables and simmer in 1" of water.
- In a skillet dry roast these spices: 1 tsp. ground cumin, ½ tsp. mustard seeds, 8 fenugreek seeds, ½ tsp. cardamom, and 1 pinch black pepper.
- Add spices to soup pot and cook for 10-15 minutes. Add sea salt to taste.
- Serve with Red Rice: in a saucepan, add 1 cup of white basmati rice with 1 ½ cups of water, ½ tsp. salt and 1 finely grated beet. Bring to a boil. Cover. Reduce heat to low and simmer for 18 minutes. Remove from heat, keep covered and let it stand for 5 minutes before serving.
- Serve with steamed seasonal vegetables drizzles with lemon juice, sea salt and pepper to taste.

Sweet Potato Soup: "Good and Vata-Pacifying"

- In a pot, bring to boil 6-7 cups of water with 4 diced sweet potatoes 2 sliced carrots, 1 bay leaf and the seeds from 1 cardamom pod. Simmer for 25-30 minutes until vegetables are soft. Add ½ tsp. salt and ¼ tsp. white pepper.
- Purée for a creamy and soothing consistency.
- Serve with roasted beets.

Water-Sautéed Vegetables

Chop 2 cups of seasonal vegetables of choice and steam.
In a skillet, dry roast ½ tsp. cumin seeds, ¼ tsp. mustard seeds, 8 fenugreek seeds. Cover with a lid and let seeds pop for a minute or two, then add ½ tsp. cardamom. Add steamed vegetables, a ¼" of water, and water sauté approximately 2-5 minutes until they are cooked to your desired texture. Keep the water boiling. Add water as needed. Salt to taste.

18 FAQ's

Phase 1 and Phase 2 Diets

Q: I'm nervous about the water intake. Won't I be living in the bathroom? I've had 3 babies and my bladder is not what it used to be!! Liquids also fill me up. How will I have room for food?

A: Dehydration is a chronic problem. Drinking 8 glasses of water per day will only replace the fluids naturally lost each day. During a cleanse we need a bit more than that.

Because we are opening the pores first with hot water and aiming to help the water absorb more efficiently, you may find that you don't have to go to the bathroom as frequently as you would think. The Rehydration Therapy techniques (see page 38) are designed so that the water doesn't run through you. Try it and see how your body reacts. That said, in all aspects of the cleanse, only do what is comfortable for you. Don't strain.

Q: Can I use coconut milk during Phase 1, in soups or other dishes?

A: As coconut milk is rich and high in fat, it does not match the low-fat guidelines. Most of the dairy milk alternatives are highly processed and not a whole food, and therefore should not be a part of the cleanse.

Q: Should I be vegetarian/vegan during the cleanse?

A: Yes, this is best. That being said, if a little lean meat - preferably chicken or turkey - will help stabilize your blood sugar and make the cleanse more comfortable, then this is a very acceptable option. This is not an endurance event.

Q: How about lemon water during Phase 1 and Phase 2?

A: Lemons will stimulate the digestive process and can be useful occasionally during the cleanse. During the Colorado Cleanse, we ask that you drink mostly plain water as its rinsing effect cannot be achieved as efficiently when anything is added to it. See Rehydration Therapy on page 38.

Q: What about tofu and tempeh during Phase 1 and Phase 2?

A: We ask that you don't do any soy during the cleanse, as it is too hard to digest and a highly allergenic food.

Q: How come no fish? Many are low-fat and it is an easy-to-digest protein.

A: The reality is that fish are unreliable in terms of toxic exposure, such as heavy metals and one of the most common allergenic foods. If you need extra protein, please read the recommendations on page 36.

Q: What kind of protein powder do you recommend?

A: It can be whey, hemp, rice, or pea, but get one with as few ingredients as possible. Concentrates are better than isolates.

Apples

Q: I get gas when I drink apple juice with my meals. Isn't that bad food combining?

A: Apple juice will have too much concentrated sugar and should be avoided. Sour, not sweet, apples are ok after a meal, or as a snack if you are crashing. Getting gas from drinking apple juice with your meal is also an indication of a very weak digestive fire and sluggish bile flow. Sour apples thin and flush the bile and are an important part of Phase 1.

Q: I have Candida and was told by my general practitioner to avoid fruits and veggies with high sugar content, such as beets and apples. What should I do instead?

A: Instead of the beets, you can have an extra glass of the Green Tonic. Malic acid is a great replacement for sour apples. Here is the protocol for taking malic acid: Stir 1-2 teaspoons into 8 oz. of water and drink up to three times daily.

Q: Can I use apple sauce instead of eating apples?

A: I recommend eating fresh apples to reap the benefits of the whole food; the apple pectin and the fresh apple's ability to thin the bile and dilate the bile ducts and the liver's biliary tubes. However, if you cannot do fresh apples, apple sauce is okay as long as it is fresh. You can also try the Emerald Apple Sauce recipe on page 116, which is a delicious raw apple sauce with parsley.

Q: Would it be all right to mix apple juice and water for my daily liquid? How about ginger and lemon?

A: Please don't add any apple juice, ginger, or lemon to the water that you're drinking between meals.

Q: If eating seasonally is a big part of this cleanse, why are we instructed to eat apples during the spring?

A: In Ayurveda, foods are classified by their qualities first. Some foods have the appropriate properties in multiple seasons. Apples are great in the spring because they are astringent and sour, and they are great in the fall because they are sweet and astringent. The astringent quality is appropriate for both seasons. During the cleanse, the apples provide malic acid that dilates the bile ducts and allows for better bile flow and liver detoxification.

Beet Tonic

Q: Directly after eating the Beet Tonic I feel good, then hours later if I eat anything else I feel nauseous and bloated on the left side, and the next morning I have really loose stools. Could this be a liver cleanse or should I stop eating the beets?

A: It is exactly that, a bile and liver flush. It is a good thing, and I would continue by eating less and slowly increasing based on your tolerance. This kind of digestive nausea has to go and should dissipate by the end of Phase 1.

Green Tonic

Q: Can I add butternut squash to the Green Tonic and use it for a larger meal?

A: Yes, in the fall and winter, you can make the Green Tonic into a satisfying soup by adding squash or other seasonal veggies. The key of a Green Tonic is for it to be made from greens. Make these variations on occasion.

Q: Can I mix my beet juice and Green Tonic together and drink it all at once? Then, skip the Beet Tonic?

A: You can mix them all together if that is easier.

Salt

Q: Should I restrict my intake of salt during the cleanse? What about Bragg's Liquid Aminos?

A: There's no need to restrict your salt intake as long as you don't feel that you consume very large quantities or need it at every meal. Be sure to use a natural Himalayan, Redmond, or Celtic Sea Salt which have natural minerals. Bragg's Aminos is soy based and is not recommended.

Oils

Q: Are all oils out? Can I use a small amount of oil as long as I keep it low-fat during Phase 1 and Phase 3?

A: Please don't add any oil to your diet during the Colorado Cleanse. Oil is concentrated and harder to digest than we want to aim for. Small amounts of healthy, food based, unprocessed fat are okay during Phase 1 and Phase 3 (main sources of these will be avocados and seeds). If you are looking for salad dressings, see the options on page 103 (fall/winter) and page 115 (spring/summer).

Q: How about flax seed oil and/or fish-oil supplements during Phase 1 and Phase 3?

A: It is preferable to avoid these. For this cleanse, get your oils naturally from the seeds, avocados, fruits and veggies.

3 Meals a Day

Q: My normal schedule is to eat breakfast around 8am, lunch (around noon), then work out after work before going home and eating dinner around 7-8pm. I will need a snack to get me through my workout. Would you recommend a snack? I've made my lunches bigger, but I don't like to feel overly full through the afternoon.

A: Yes, the big lunches will help, as will more water in the afternoon. Most workouts don't require a snack unless it is very long. A bigger lunch, if the digestive fire is optimal, will last you with more energy into the workout. Remember, as your blood sugar balances and you become an even better fat burner, your need for a snack will slowly disappear. If you need a snack, eat an apple.

Morning Ghee

Q: Why is ghee better than other oils, such as olive oil, coconut oil or sesame oil?

A: Ghee has unique properties, and that is why it has been the oleation agent of choice for so many thousands of years:
- Ghee is balancing for all body types during all seasons.
- It cools the body while strengthening the digestion.
- It reduces acidity in the digestion and in the tissues.
- Its light nature (low saturated fat content) makes it easy to digest and allows the fatty acids to penetrate the deep tissues, deeply and thoroughly lubricating them.
- Ghee also acts as a carrier for nutrients to be carried across the gut wall and chelate toxins to be removed from the cells, while other oils are too heavy for this.
- See Chapter 11 for more information on the benefits of ghee.

As I mention in chapter 11, if you are vegan, cannot tolerate the taste of ghee, or need an alternative for any other reason, flax seed oil and olive oil are acceptable alternatives. Though coconut oil has many health benefits, it is a medium chain fatty acid that is not broken down by bile from the liver and gallbladder because it is already a smaller (pre-digested) fatty acid than 97% of dietary fats which are long chain fatty acids. As a result coconut oil will not purge the gallbladder like ghee would and there for is not the best choice to replace the ghee in the main cleanse. That said, folks without a gallbladder or a severe difficulty digesting fats can use coconut oil instead of ghee in the main cleanse because it would not strain the liver and gallbladder and it does offer all the other benefits that we gain from using the ghee.

Q. Why do we increase the dosage of ghee every day and how does that work in the body?

A: If we take too much ghee too soon, we can overwhelm the gallbladder. So we slowly exercise the gallbladder by flushing it with higher doses of ghee each day. The last day of Phase 2 is a big flush with ghee in the AM ending with the Final Flush in the PM. I have some video newsletters about the need to flush the bile that may be helpful. Please see my free articles online:
- Surprising Symptoms of Digestion (lifespa.com/digestivehealth)
- Most Important ½ Inch of Your Body (lifespa.com/skin)
- The Miracle of Lymph (lifespa.com/lymph)

Q: Is the ghee protocol still the same for someone without a gallbladder?

A: It is based on your comfort. Take only 2 - 3 teaspoons of ghee each morning. Do not increase the ghee. This is a safe amount that will be enough to help you enter fat metabolism and get the bile to flow.

Q: Does ghee (a saturated fat) raise the LDL cholesterol and triglyceride levels?

A: Yes, ghee alone will raise your cholesterol if it is taken at high dosages for a long period of time. But at the correct dose, ghee will lower LDL. During Phase 2, we are eating a nonfat diet while taking the ghee for only these seven days. After taking the ghee each morning, the body is naturally forced into fat metabolism mode which not only removes the ghee from the body but the toxic fat-soluble chemicals stored in the fat cells as well. Though a blood test administered during Phase 2 may show temporarily increased cholesterol levels, studies show that this process ultimately lowers cholesterol.

Q: I am having significant diarrhea today. The diarrhea takes a few hours after the ghee to set in. Can I keep up the ghee? Should I give it one more day?

A: If the loose stools are uncomfortable then back off the ghee to a dose that makes it tolerable. The key is comfort and your stamina.

Also, stop the Liver Repair for a few days and see if this helps. This formula is a bile flusher that can sometimes cause too much bile in the gut and loosen the stool.

Q: Why don't we take the Warm Digest or Cool Digest before the ghee?

A: If you feel you need it to digest the ghee, you can. But because we are resetting the digestive fire in Phase 3, and preparing the digestion in Phase 1, it is not necessary to take the Warm Digest or Cool Digest with the ghee.

Q: Can I eat the ghee without melting it?

A: Yes, you can eat ghee without melting it if you find it palatable. Enjoy it right off the spoon. Bon appetite!

Kitchari

Q: Can I use brown rice instead of white rice in the kitchari?

A: Brown rice does have more nutrients, but holds more toxins and impurities in the husk than white rice, which has had the husk removed. Brown rice also requires more digestive fire to break down the husk. During the cleanse we are trying to take the stress off digestion by eating easy-to-digest food – baby food really – in order to heal and repair the gut during Phase 2. The white rice is actually quite nutritious, easy to digest and ideal for the purposes of this cleanse.
If you would like more fiber and protein and/or are having trouble digesting the white rice, you can try substituting with quinoa.

Rehydration Therapy

Q: I'm hot all the time (pitta, perimenopause). Does it have to be hot water?

A: Please give the Hot Sips a try. As it rehydrates you and stimulates lymph flow, your body will dissipate the heat much better. This, along with your Daily Ounces, will be the best rehydration technique, as well as the best way to help your body remove the excess heat.

Q: Can I have herbal teas between meals?

A: It is best to have herbal teas with meals. It is ideal to sip plain warm-to-hot water as much as possible between meals because it is more hydrating and detoxifying for the lymphatic system.

Q: Can I drink ice water?

A: Please avoid ice water during this cleanse. Ice water constricts the vessels of the circulatory system and compromises hydration and the lymphatic system, which can slow down digestion and release of toxins.

Q: I understand the concept of sipping more warm to hot water on the cleanse, but doesn't too much water cool or even extinguish digestive fire and thin digestive juices?

A: This large amount of water will certainly dilute digestive juices if taken with the meal. Instead, try sipping some hot water with the meal and drinking a large glass of water 15-20 minutes before the meal and in between meals - but not during the meal.

Q: I am having to get up multiple times during the night to use the bathroom after drinking so much water all day. I am losing sleep. Any recommendations?

A: Try to get most of the water in during the day and stop drinking at 6 or 7pm.

Exercise

Q: I have been doing a lot of endurance training. Normally I would take a Cliff bar and maybe a GU packet to prevent a bonk on a 2-7 hour bike ride. During the cleanse, what can I use to replenish those carbs when I need to be fueled up?

A: During Phase 2, I would suggest backing off on the endurance training and doing the workout I suggest in Chapter 6. During a cleanse you need to rest the body, or the detox will not get as deep. Even during Phase 1 and Phase 3, I suggest shorter workouts like the yoga and 12-Minute Workout I outlined. You are being nudged into a fat burning detox state - not an endurance state. Ultimately, the rest period will enhance your performance.

Yoga

Q: I currently practice yoga at home. Should I stick with my current practice/poses, try the Sun Salutations in this book, do Dr. John's yoga poses in the Ayurveda for Detox DVD?

A: The poses in the Ayurveda for Detox DVD are a different from the Sun Salutations detailed in this book, and are especially designed to support detox and stimulate the flow of prana and lymph. The long holds will help enhance normal physiological function as well as help release old mental and emotional patterns. The Sun Salutations on page 51 of this book accomplish these same goals. You can also choose to practice your own routine and incorporate longer holds. 10 breaths for each pose is a good guideline. If you cannot hold a pose for that long, that pose may be too strenuous for the Colorado Cleanse.

Q: I woke up this morning feeling pretty achy, particularly in my hips and thighs. When I did the yoga practice I really felt discomfort in my thighs and particularly in my hamstrings. Can you suggest why this is happening?

A: It may take a couple of days for your body to get used to the yoga. This could also be due to a cleansing effect. Be gentle with yourself and don't push too hard. As we start Phase 2, you should begin to feel lighter. The Abhyanga self-massage and an Epsom salt bath can be excellent sources of relief for soreness.

Abhyanga Self-Massage

Q: Is it necessary to keep the oil on my body or can I wash it off (especially my head and hair) and follow my usual moisturizing routine? It's very greasy, and I'm afraid it will stain my towel and clothes.

A: It is not necessary to keep the oil on the hair and body. I suggest doing the massage at the end of a shower with the water running. This way you will use just a very small amount of oil with the water to help disperse it, gently rinse and towel dry. A small film of oil will be left but it will not be greasy and should not stain.

Q: You mention oiling the head as part of the daily self-massage. Does that mean I have to wash my hair every day to get the oil out?

A: It is optional to put the oil on your hair. If you do, try to get it into the scalp and not so much on the ends. When shampooing, clean the ends of the hair but don't try to get all the oil from the scalp out until the cleanse is done. If you need to be presentable during the day then oiling the hair is optional.

Self–Inquiry

Q: What can I expect as the emotional toxins are released from my body?

A: When the emotional toxins are released, it manifests as more clarity. You just become more aware of why you do what you do emotionally. The idea isn't to be dragged through the emotional mud. With heightened awareness, you will be more clear, and therefore be able to engage in transformational action steps that will free you from reacting to old negative emotional patterns.

Caffeine and Nicotine Detox

Q: Can I drink coffee on the cleanse? Is it really that bad for me?

A: If you are addicted to coffee, this a great time to break the habit if you are up for it. With the cleanse, the bile will be flowing and this will be the easiest time to do it. If you cannot, then do your best to cut back. Drink 8 oz. of water before and after each cup. Try to have it with meals and not on an empty stomach. Brewing it with cardamom also helps protect the gut and neutralize the caffeine. Green tea is a good replacement while you are weaning off, but read my comments on tea below. Good luck!

Q: Is it okay to have a cup of organic decaf coffee during the cleanse?

A: No, decaf coffee is more dehydrating than regular coffee and it still has caffeine. The key to Phase 2 is to heal the gut and this would defeat the purpose. It is best to not have caffeine during the cleanse.

Q: Is Black Tea or Green Tea okay?

A: It is best to not drink caffeine, but if you are addicted they are much better than coffee and not irritating to the bowel. If you feel like you can't get through your day without caffeinated tea, that may mean you are exhausted and using the tea to stimulate your body to make energy you don't have. Focus on weaning off by drinking one cup of water before and after your tea and gradually using tea with less and less caffeine. If you are going to have caffeinated tea, have it with food - preferably at lunch - rather than on an empty stomach.

Q: I am a smoker. What can I do during the cleanse to help me cut down and/or quit?

A: This is a great time to make this happen! Smoking is a nervous system stimulant that we become addicted to. When you go into fat burning during the Colorado Cleanse, you will be burning calm fuel which will allow you a window to reset the nervous system to function without stimulants. Here are some tips to ease the transition:

- Suck on cardamom pods and fennel seeds throughout the day to help relieve cravings.
- Practice the One Minute Meditation (page 54) 5 – 10 times a day or as needed, especially when you are caught in a nicotine craving.
- Take 2-3 capsules of LifeSpa's Anxiety-Free formula 3 times per day with meals.

Q: I love chocolate and eat it every day. I've read it has amazing health benefits. Can I eat it during the cleanse and, if not, what are some tips to wean off?

A: Chocolate contains caffeine, as well as an interesting blend of other natural chemicals – some stimulants, others not – that are not conducive to the cleanse. Please avoid it for these two weeks, and use the tips on detoxing from coffee, above, if you are having a hard time. Read more about the health benefits and components of chocolate in my article, The Chocolate Effect, at lifespa.com/chocolate

Cleansing/Detox Symptoms

Q: What possible detox reactions could we experience during this cleanse?

A: This is a tough question.   As we are all so different I can't say what uncomfortable things to expect. Hopefully it is all good. Whatever we do experience is definitely a symptom of what may be an underlying imbalance. The problems we experience during the cleanse are VERY diagnostic and can be useful to treat an underlying problem that may have been hiding for years. There are some very common experiences – such as days of fatigue and irritability, mild muscle aches – which are signs of cleansing. Many of us also have gut and digestive problems that show up during Phase 2 and will be treated during Phase 3.

Q: Wow, I feel horrible today. I am just trying to understand if this feeling is from toxins being released or from not having enough food. Hard to know if it's blood sugar related or just those emotions being released. Is anyone else struggling? Are we supposed to have these down days or are we are supposed to feel good the whole time?

A: Up days are common and so are down days. This could be from toxins releasing. If so, drinking more water will help. This could also be from emotions releasing. Try practicing random acts of kindness, even though you may have no desire to do so. Also, make sure you are getting enough protein. See the recommendations for blood sugar balancing on page 36. You can also stop the herbs for a couple of days and eat more from the Rejuvenate or Nourish meal options.

Q: My skin and mucous membranes are still feeling very dry from the low-fat and nonfat diets, in spite of the all the Morning Ghee and all the water that I've been drinking.

A: This means there's a significant level of dehydration, which means your intestinal inner skin is dry as well.   Read my video-newsletter about how inner skin determines what outer skin looks like at lifespa.com/skin

Q: My husband and I have been feeling hot in the evenings at dinnertime and after, especially feeling flushed in the face. Is this anything to do with the cleanse? I have some pitta imbalance, could it be due to that?

A: Yes, this could be due to a pitta imbalance. As we enter Phase 2 this should even out. Focus on eating plenty of greens and doing the best you can with the Rehydration Therapy. If it persists, try stopping the herbs for a couple of days. If you improve, restart the herbs with just 1 capsule of each herb per day. Stopping the Beet Tonics may help as well.

Q: Each day after lunch I've gotten very gassy.

A: When we start such a high fiber diet, we begin to scrub the intestinal villi, which can cause some digestive disturbance. When we start Phase 2 we will stop the high fiber diet and start to heal the now cleansed intestinal villi. The gut should feel soothed by the kitchari diet.

Q: I vomited during Phase 1. Am I on the wrong track?

A: If you are experiencing nausea or if you regurgitate your food, this is a sign of bile flow issues that probably should be addressed. Over time this issue will affect the ability to digest wheat, dairy and other foods. Please read my article "Gallbladder Health Food and Recipes" (lifespa.com/GB). In the meantime, you can follow the Nourish meal option, reduce the dose of ghee to 2-3 teaspoons each day, and stop all the herbs. Once you feel better, you can restart the herbs, beginning with 1 capsule, 1 time per day. To relieve nausea symptoms, take 1 teaspoon of baking soda in 1 cup of warm water.

Q: I am experiencing low back pain during Phase 1. What can this be and what can I do?

A: This is quite common and often due to the process of kidney detox. Make sure to get your Daily Ounces and get enough protein in your meals. Consider adding a small protein powder smoothie or lean chicken to your meals. To relieve the back pain, take a hot Epsom salt bath. For maintenance, incorporate the Abhyanga self-massage and yoga practices daily (see chapter 7).

Low Blood Sugar

(Please read the FAQs on kitchari on page 133 for more information on blood sugar).

Q: What are the symptoms of unstable blood sugar?

A: A simple test for checking your blood sugar, other than a blood test, is to see if you can comfortably make it through the day with only 3 meals and no snacks. If you can do this without a craving, mood swings, need for a nap or a snack, the blood sugar is likely okay. If you sense that your blood sugar is unstable:
- Eat 4 meals a day during the cleanse.
- Stick with the Rejuvenate or Nourish meal option during the Main Cleanse, adding low-fat protein if needed.
- Increase the Regenerate, Sugar Destroyer and Beet Cleanse dosage to 2 or 3 capsules with each meal.
- Focus on getting adequate protein at every meal.

Q: Can I use natural sweeteners like agave, brown rice syrup, raw honey, coconut sugar or barley malt during the cleanse?

A: No, please stay away from all sweeteners during the cleanse.

Q: How about stevia?

A: Although stevia does not affect the blood sugar the way other sweeteners do, I recommend staying away from it during the cleanse to give your body a chance to detox from the sweet taste. Even if we work hard to balance the blood sugar during the cleanse, a lingering addiction to the sweet taste can undermine lasting results.

Occasional Acid Reflux and Heartburn

Q: I sometimes have heartburn, which must mean I have too much digestive fire. Won't turning it back on make these symptoms worse?

A: Actually, acid issues may be caused either by too much or too little digestive fire. You can read more about this and find out how to test the cause in my article, Cool Your Digestion (lifespa.com/heartburn1). Turning on the digestive fire is more of a calibration for the digestive strength and will help either way.

Q: I've been getting heartburn lately, especially when drinking the hot water. Is heartburn part of the cleanse? Should I stop drinking the hot water?

A: No this is not part of the cleanse. Remember we are only sipping the hot water every 10-15 minutes, just 2-3 sips each time. Try taking 2 capsules of Cool Digest before each meal.

Edema

Q: I'm finding that I'm retaining water in my legs and have a bit of edema. Is this normal? And what can I do to alleviate it?

A: This is a sign of some underlying lymph sluggishness. Hot water and Manjistha can be increased. Increase Manjistha to 3 capsules, 3 times a day and sip more hot water. Try doing the self-massage towards the heart twice a day and make sure you are exercising. If the edema persists, stop the cleanse and see your medical doctor.

Headaches

Q: Do you expect that some people may get headaches on this cleanse? If so, do you have any advice for relief? I want to avoid migraines.

A: Actually, because we are preparing the detox channels and balancing blood sugar with Phase 1 before we start Phase 2, headaches are uncommon unless one is not hydrated - which you can remedy with the Rehydration Therapy in chapter 4 - or if they are detoxing from something like coffee, chocolate or cigarettes. In this case, you can place a cool ice cloth on the forehead and a hot water bottle on the feet for 20-30 minutes. This is an amazing technique to help remove detox withdrawal symptoms. Also, read the FAQs regarding low blood sugar, which may need more attention (page 138).

Q: Is one small bowel movement a day normal during Phase 2?

A: Yes, this is perfectly normal. If it becomes uncomfortable, use an herbal formula like Triphala or Elim I to keep things moving.

Insomnia

Q: Falling asleep is difficult and I have been consistently waking up at 3 or 4 am. I need sleep! What could be causing this?

A: When the body is actively detoxifying, the liver becomes very active between 10pm and 2am. This stimulation can keep some folks up. One trick is to get to bed early and not wait until 10 or 11pm to attempt sleep. I also use an herbal formula called Brahmi Brain, which boosts the body's energy enough to put itself to sleep at night and cools the liver. Please read more about this in my article, "Sleep Support" (lifespa.com/SleepSupport). Blood sugar may also play a role. Please read the section below for suggestions to stabilize blood sugar.

Nauseous

Q: I am nauseated and having loose stools today. What else can I do to ease my discomfort?

A: Cut back on the Liver Repair to only 1 capsule a day. After a few days, add back 1 capsule at a time until you find the dose that is right for you. If you are in Phase 2, take less ghee – 2-3 teaspoons – for a day or two.

Tired

Q: I feel exhausted and fatigued during Phase 2. Should I stop?

A: If you feel weak, dizzy or hungry on any of the meal options, add some lean chicken or a nonfat protein drink to your meals to bring your blood sugar into balance. Do not hesitate on this. If your blood sugar crashes, your body stops burning fat, which is where toxins are stored. Each time you do this cleanse your ability to use your fat as an energy source will improve, your blood sugar will balance.

Q: I feel very foggy and dissociated from my body. Definitely not as mentally sharp as usual. Is this normal?

A: When you are detoxing during the cleanse, two things are happening. First, you are burning more fat so you are more calm and mellow. In the fat are stored fat-soluble toxins that are being flushed into the blood and liver for elimination. Imagine cleaning a pool – initially it looks pretty bad, but soon when the toxins are flushed the water clears, as does the mental clarity.

Weight Gain

Q: I am gaining weight on this cleanse, and wondering what to do about that. I am doing most of my normal level of activity and training, though feeling really sluggish during exercise.

A: I see three possible reasons for this:
- Stress – Sometimes the body will not let the fat go until it is convinced the war is over. If life is very stressful, this may be a cause. Try focusing more on all the Optional Stress-Relief Practices in chapter 7, particularly yoga and meditation, and make sure you are getting enough sleep. All of these will help create a feeling of relaxation and calm, reassuring your body that the stress is over and it can let go of the fat.
- Slow digestion – you may need Triphala or Elim I to encourage elimination. Take 2-4 capsules, twice a day, on an empty stomach with 8 oz. of water.
- Unstable blood sugar – Please read the blood sugar balancing recommendations on page 36.

Q: Am I supposed to be losing weight as the fat burns? I am following all the protocols, but not necessarily shedding weight. How do I make sure I am burning fat to detox?

A: Weight loss is not the only determining factor if your body is burning fat. Weight is also affected by the lymph. If you find yourself less hungry and able to move through the day with 3 meals and no snacks and a steady supply of calm energy, you are burning fat.
Remember, this cleanse is not a weight loss boot camp. If we follow the Integration plan in chapter 16, we will continue to naturally lose pounds until we reach our ideal weight (according to our bodies, not our minds).

Q: When the massage oil gets absorbed, does it interfere with fat metabolism? Or are the inside and outside oleation processes not connected at all?

A: The external oleation won't affect fat metabolism. The oil on the outside of the skin acts more as a carrier for the herbs in the oil to penetrate the cell wall than a source of fat for the body.
External massage will oleate the intercellular tissue where the lymph drains waste, allowing for the drainage and removal of this waste to be more efficient.

Weight Loss – Too Much

Q: I am afraid I will lose too much weight, especially during Phase 2, as I am already a little too thin.

A: If you are concerned about losing weight:

- Decrease all herbs to only 1 capsule per day with your main meal (lunch).
- Eat 4 meals per day throughout the cleanse and eat your food in a relaxed manner.
- Eat more avocado and seeds during Phase 1 and Phase 3.
- Follow the Nourish meal option during Phase 2.
- Cut the ghee back to 2–3 teaspoons each morning during Phase 2.

Constipation

Top 7 strategies for relieving constipation:

- Take LifeSpa's Elim I herbal formula (see protocol directly below).
  An alternative to Elim I is Triphala, which you can find at most health food stores. Alternatively, cook prunes into your kitchari.
- During Phase 1 and Phase 3, (not Phase 2) take some chia seeds after meals. Take 1 Tablespoon of chia seeds in 8 oz. of water, stir and let sit for 1-2 minutes, then drink.
- Make sure you are following the Rehydration Therapy protocol on page 38.
- Follow the yoga protocol every day to tone and massage the abdominal region.
- Eat an light, early dinner.
- Be sure you are eating enough fiber in the form of steamed vegetables. During Phase 1 and Phase 3, eat the Beet Tonic and Green Tonic every day, in addition to any vegetables on the appropriate Seasonal Cleansing Foods list in Appendix 2 of this book.
- Increase the dosages of Beet Cleanse and Liver Repair to 2 capsules of each with each meal.

Elim I Protocol:

Start by taking 2 capsules first thing in the morning, before the ghee if you are in Phase 2, and 2 capsules before bed at night.

- If you do not move your bowels early the next day, take 3 capsules each in the AM and PM.

- Continue increasing daily until you start eliminating once a day in the morning. The maximum dose is 6 capsules in the AM and 6 capsules in the PM.

- Once you start eliminating 1-2 times per day, stay at your current dose in the AM and PM for a two week period.

- Slowly wean off: after two weeks, if elimination is steady at once in the morning, gradually reduce the dosage by 1 capsule in the AM and PM for two more weeks.

- Continue decreasing your dosage by 1 capsule in the AM and PM every two weeks.

- If you become constipated again, increase to the previous dose for 2 weeks. Once you are eliminating once in the morning again, start decreasing your dosage.

Q: Can we do enemas or colonics during the cleanse?

A: I'm not a big fan of every day enemas. But if you think you need it on a given day, go ahead and do that. I would suggest a ¼ cup retention enema with cold-pressed sesame oil (warm the oil to body temperature first). You can also follow the Elim I protocol above to help keep the bowels moving. Make sure you are sipping warm to hot water every 15 minutes.
Colonics can become habit forming. As part of a cleanse in the early stages, it can be ok. But after the cleanse we are resetting digestion and elimination, and a colonic will alter this.

Q: Can I take a natural laxative to relieve constipation, like senna or cascara sagrada?

A: These herbal laxatives are bowel irritants that can irritate, dehydrate and desensitize the intestinal mucosa. Though they will get you to go, they are habit forming and problematic. Remember, our goal is to heal the villi, not irritate them, so use these laxatives as a last resort. Magnesium is better but still dehydrates the bowel. Use senna tea if necessary as a temporary fix. Learn more at lifespa. com/constipation

Final Flush

Q: I have to work early/travel on day 12. Should I do the Final Flush on a different day?

A: If you have to wake up early the next morning and go somewhere, do the laxative earlier in the evening or do the laxative a day earlier or a day later. If you do it a day later, stick to the diet during that extra day but don't do the ghee.

Q: Is the laxative going to be very uncomfortable? What should I expect?
A: You will have 3 - 10 loose bowel movements. There may be some cramping in your belly, but you will feel lighter and cleaner. The ghee has moved toxins to your lymph, which has brought them to your digestion via the liver. The laxative will help clear all these toxins out. If you are very sensitive, use the prune juice.

Q: Should I take some electrolytes the morning after the laxative therapy?

A: Normally, this is not necessary unless the loose stools persist for a couple of days which is extremely uncommon.

Q: Last time I did the cleanse, I did not have a laxative effect. What can I do this time to ensure I get the full benefit?

A: If the Final Flush does not work for you that night, you can take another dose of the laxative therapy that next morning or the next night. If you have been having loose stools throughout the cleanse, it may be that your bowels just don't have that much to eliminate, in which case you can rest assured that you have been eliminating the toxins that have been building up in your digestive tract throughout the cleanse.

Q: The Colorado Cleanse used to use castor oil. Why not anymore?

A: Castor oil is made from the castor bean or seed. The raw seed contains a toxic protein called ricin which is denatured and inactivated when heated and pressed into castor oil. However, harvesting the seed/bean exposes the pickers to the toxic ricin.

This has become a health issue for the growers who can experience permanent nerve damage from the ricin exposure on the surface of the plant. Because processing of castor oil has become a human health risk for workers, we at LifeSpa have chosen not to use castor oil for our cleanses.

Integration

Q: I worry that I will completely fall prey to cake, cookies, ice cream, etc. after a restrictive diet. It seems that once I allow myself a small treat, I quickly fall into a sugar trap & want it all the time!

A: The nice part of the Colorado Cleanse is that the re-entry is built into the cleanse via Phase 3. In Phase 3, we reset the digestive fire so that you can digest and break down more difficult foods. Thus you assimilate nutrients better and be more satisfied from eating healthier food, and not feel the need to binge. Most cleanses starve you and don't strengthen your digestion so you are left hungry and dangerous! After Phase 3, follow the Integration plan in Chapter 16 to reintegrate into a non-cleanse routine and create lasting benefits. If you deviate once in a while, don't worry! What matters is what you do most of the time, not the occasional slip-ups.

Q: I'm surprised by how quickly I feel bad with the few times I've "cheated" on this cleanse. Why is that? I would hate to think that the only way to feel healthy is to have a restricted diet forever.

A: The last thing this cleanse sets out to do is to leave you on a restricted diet. The goal is to prepare the body to detox normally and digest an array of foods by resetting good digestive function. Be sure to follow the digestive reset protocol closely during Phase 3 to get the full benefit.

The reason you may feel bad when you cheat during Phase 2 is because you are in villi-healing mode and eating a very easy-to-digest diet. During this process the villi become very vulnerable and exposed. If you eat something harder to digest before properly resetting digestion with Phase 3, you will irritate the villi, which can potentially cause stomach upset and malaise.

Q: If we are in situations (traveling, vacation, visiting people) where we cannot keep to the current seasonal diet during the Integration weeks, is it devastating to eat some other foods once in a while? And then return to the current seasonal diet as soon as possible?

A: No it will not be devastating at all, though I would suggest that in the weeks directly following the cleanse, you continue with the current seasonal diet as much as possible in order to allow the villi to heal. Be sure to take your digestive formula, Warm Digest or Cool Digest with you and take some before a large heavy meal to facilitate digestion.

Other

Q: I am menstruating. Should I make any adjustments to the cleanse?

A: If you are feeling good and strong, you do not need to make any adjustments to the cleanse. If you don't feel strong, don't increase the ghee dosages during Phase 2 and stick with 2-3 teaspoons a day. As always, listen to your body.

Q: I binged. What did I do wrong?

A: We always say if you are straining during the cleanse you will not burn fat as well. You may start craving, and you may want to binge. In the beginning of each section of the Day-by-Day Guide on pages 18-31, we give strategies to slow down the intensity of the cleanse. It is never a disaster when this happens - just pick up where you left off and, this time around, don't strain.

Q: Should probiotics be discontinued during the cleanse? How about multi-vitamins/ minerals?

A: I do suggest stopping all supplements during the cleanse except your medications and the cleanse herbs. You can go back on them as soon as you are finished with Phase 3. That said, if there are one or two supplements that you can't live without, go ahead and take them. The key is to not overwhelm the digestive system during the cleanse but to give it a chance to heal before we amp up the digestive fire again.

Q: I work the night shift. Do you have any suggestions for how to make this cleanse work on a night shift schedule?

A: For the night shift, just switch it around. Make the meal when you wake up around midday your main meal and then have two other ones early evening and middle of the night. Try to stick with 3 meals a day (in this case, night) with no snacks and you will be fine.

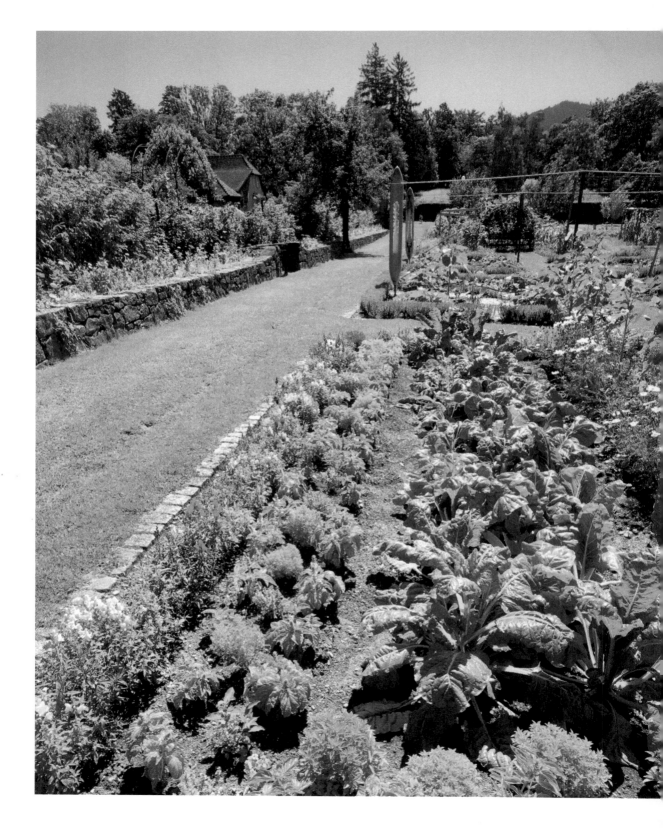

Appendix

Appendix 1
Foods to Avoid During the Cleanse

Dairy
Butter
Cheese
Cottage cheese
Lactose
Milk
Whey
Yogurt

Caffeine
Black Tea
Coffee
Green Tea

Chocolate

Corn
(Fresh corn is fine)
Cornmeal
Corn Syrup
Grits
High-Fructose Corn Syrup
Hominy
Polenta
Popcorn

Eggs
Including egg whites

Fermented Foods
Kombucha
Pickles
Sauerkraut
Vinegar

Modified Foods (GM)
To avoid GM foods, choose organic or foods with a clear non-GM label on the front.
Animal feed *(thus meat, eggs, dairy)*
Corn
Golden rice
Oils *(especially cotton seed, canola and rapeseed.)*
Potatoes
Salmon
Soy
Squash
Sugar Beets
Tomatoes

Grain Products
(Even if Gluten-Free)
Bread
Crackers
Noodles
Pasta
Tortillas

Gluten
Barley
Bulgur
Couscous
Durum
Einkorn
Kamut
Malt
Oats (*except for oats that specify "not contaminated with wheat" or "Certified Gluten-Free"*)
Semolina
Spelt
Triticale
Rye
Wheat
Wheat bran
Wheat germ
Wheat starch

Nicotine

Meats
Beef
Duck
Deli Meats (*Cold Cuts*)
Lamb
Pork
Venison

Nuts
All nuts

Oils
All oils

Processed Foods
Eat only whole grains, legumes, vegetables, fruits and lean meat.

Peanuts

Seafood
Fish
Shellfish

Soy
Edamame
Miso
Soy milk
Soy protein powder
Tempeh
Texturized Vegetable Protein
Tofu

Sweeteners
Artificial sweeteners
Corn Syrup
Fructose
Glucose
High-Fructose Corn Syrup
Honey
Low- or no-cal sweeteners
Maple Syrup
Sugar

Table Salt

Appendix 2
Spring Cleansing Foods (March–June)

- Though these are not the only items you can eat, they are the most beneficial foods for cleansing during the spring.
- An asterisk (*) means that this food is particularly balancing during the springtime.
- To see a complete list of seasonal foods to enjoy when you are not cleansing (please visit lifespa.com/eatseasonally).

VEGETABLES
*Alfalfa Sprouts
Artichokes
*Asparagus
*Bean Sprouts
Beets
*Bell Peppers
*Bitter Melon
Broccoli
*Brussels Sprouts
*Cabbage
*Carrots
*Cauliflower
*Celery
*Chicory
*Chilies *(dried)*
Cilantro
*Collard Greens
*Corn
*Dandelion
*Endive
Fennel
*Garlic
Ginger
*Green Beans
*Hot Peppers
Jicama
*Kale
Leeks
*Lettuce
*Mushrooms
*Mustard Greens
*Onions
*Parsley
*Peas
*Potatoes (baked)
*Radishes
Seaweed
Snow Peas
*Spinach
*Swiss Chard
*Turnips
*Watercress

FRUIT
Eat separately - do not combine with other foods. Eat sweet fruits separately from sour fruits.
Sweet Fruits
Papayas
Sour Fruits
Sour Apples
Blueberries
Grapefruit
Lemons
Limes
Pomegranates
Raspberries
Strawberries
Other Berries

LEGUMES
*All Sprouted Beans
Small Beans
Small beans are easier to digest than large beans.

Adzuki
Black Gram
*Lentils
*Mung
Split Pea
Large Beans
Black
Black Eyed Peas
Cannellini
Garbanzo
Fava
*Kidney
*Lima
Navy
Pinto

GRAINS

Amaranth
Buckwheat
Millet
Oats *(gluten-free)*
Quinoa
Rice, Brown
    (long grain)
Rice, White
    (long grain)

SPICES

Anise
Asafoetida
Basil
Bay Leaf
*Black Pepper
Chamomile
Caraway

Cardamom
*Cayenne
Cinnamon
*Clove
Coriander
Cumin
Dill
Fennel
Fenugreek
Garlic
Ginger
Horseradish
Marjoram
Mustard
Nutmeg
Oregano
Peppermint
Poppy Seeds
Rosemary
Saffron
Sage
Spearmint
Thyme
Turmeric

SEEDS

*Only during
Phase 1 and 2.*
Chia
Flax
Hemp
Pine Nuts
Pumpkin
Sesame
Sunflower

LEAN MEAT

*If needed to stabilize
blood sugar.*
Chicken *(white)*
Turkey *(white)*

BEVERAGES

Plain Water
    (room temp - hot)

HERB TEA

*Optional,
with meals.*
Alfalfa
*Cardamom
*Chicory
*Cinnamon
*Cloves
*Dandelion
*Hibiscus
*Orange Peel
*Strawberry Leaf

Summer Cleansing Foods (July–Oct)

- Though these are not the only items you can eat, they are the most beneficial foods for cleansing during the summer and fall.
- An asterisk (*) means that this food is particularly balancing during the summertime.
- To see a complete list of seasonal foods to enjoy when you are not cleansing (please visit lifespa.com/eatseasonally).

VEGETABLES
Alfalfa Sprouts
*Artichokes
*Asparagus
Bean Sprouts
*Beet greens
*Bell Peppers
*Bitter Melon
*Broccoli
*Cabbage
*Cauliflower
*Celery
Chicory
*Cilantro
Collard Greens
Corn
*Cucumbers
*Dandelion
Eggplant
Endive
*Fennel
Green Beans
*Jicama
*Kale
*Lettuce
Mushrooms

Mustard Greens
*Okra
Parsley
Peas
Pumpkin
*Radishes (modertion)
*Seaweed
*Snow Peas
Spinach (moderation)
*Acorn Squash
Winter Squash
Sweet Potatoes
Swiss Chard
Tomatoes (sweet)
Turnip Greens
*Watercress
*Zucchini

LEGUMES
All Bean Sprouts
Small Beans
Small beans are easier to digest than large beans.
  *Adzuki
  *Black Gram
  Lentils
  *Mung
  *Split Pea
Large Beans
  Black
  Black Eyed Peas
  Cannellini
  Garbanzo
  Fava
  *Kidney
  *Lima
  Navy
  Pinto

FRUIT
Eat separately - do not combine with other foods.
Eat sweet fruits separately from sour fruits.
Eat melons by themselves.

Sweet Fruits
  *Apricots
  *Cherries *(ripe)*
  Figs
  *Grapes
  *Mangoes
  Nectarines
  Papayas *(small amounts)*
  *Peaches *(ripe, peeled)*
  *Pears
  *Persimmons

Sour Fruits
  *Sour Apples
  *Blueberries
  *Cranberries
  *Guavas
  Oranges
  *Pineapple
  *Plums (ripe)
  *Pomegranates
  *Raspberries
  *Strawberries
  Tangerines
  Melons
  *Cantaloupe
  *Melon (all)

SPICES
Anise
Asafoetida
*Chamomile
*Coriander
Cumin
Fennel
Peppermint
Saffron
Spearmint

SEEDS
Only during Phase 1 and 2.
Chia
Flax
Hemp
*Pumpkin
Sesame
*Sunflower

LEAN MEAT
If needed to stabilize blood sugar.
Chicken *(white)*
Turkey *(white)*

BEVERAGES
Plain Water
(room temp - hot)

GRAINS
Oats *(gluten-free)*
Rice *(brown or white)*
Quinoa

HERB TEA
Optional, with meals.
*Chicory
*Dandelion
*Hibiscus
*Mint

Winter Cleansing Foods (Nov–Feb)

- Though these are not the only items you can eat, they are the most beneficial foods for cleansing during the winter.
- An asterisk (*) means that this food is particularly balancing during the wintertime.
- To see a complete list of seasonal foods to enjoy when you are not cleansing (please visit lifespa.com/eatseasonally).

VEGETABLES
Artichokes Hearts
*Beets
*Brussels Sprouts
*Carrots
*Chilies
Corn
Fennel
Eggplant *(cooked)*
*Garlic
Ginger
Hot Peppers
Leeks
Okra
Onions
Parsley
Potatoes *(mashed)*
*Pumpkins
Seaweed *(cooked)*
Acorn Squash
*Winter Squash
*Sweet Potatoes
*Tomatoes
Turnips

LEGUMES
Mung *(split, yellow)*
Red Lentils

GRAINS
*Amaranth
Buckwheat *(moderation)*
Millet *(moderation)*
*Oats *(gluten-free)*
*Quinoa
Rice *(white)*
*Rice *(brown)*

FRUIT
Eat separately - do not combine with other foods. Eat sweet fruits separately from sour fruits. Eat melons by themselves.

Sweet Fruits
Apricots
*Bananas
Coconuts *(ripe)*
*Figs
*Grapes

*Mangoes
Nectarines
*Papayas
Peaches
Pears *(ripe)*
*Persimmons

Sour Fruits
Sour Apples
Blueberries
Cherries
Cranberries *(cooked)*
*Grapefruit
Guava
*Lemons
*Limes
*Oranges
Pineapples
Plums
Strawberries
*Tangerines
Melons
Cantaloupe *(with lemon)*

SPICES

*Anise
*Asafetida
*Basil
Bay Leaf
*Black Pepper
Caraway
*Cardamom
Cayenne
Chamomile
*Cinnamon
Clove
Coriander
*Cumin
Dill
*Fennel
Fenugreek
Garlic
*Ginger
Horseradish
Marjoram
Mustard
Nutmeg
Oregano
Peppermint
Poppy Seeds
Rosemary
*Saffron
Sage
Spearmint
Thyme
*Turmeric

SEEDS

*Only during
Phase 1 and 2.*

Chia
Flax
Hemp
Pine Nuts
Pumpkin
Sesame
Sunflower

LEAN MEAT

*If needed to stabilize
blood sugar.*

Chicken *(white)*
Turkey *(white)*

BEVERAGES

Plain Water
(room temp - hot)

HERB TEAS

*Optional,
with meals.*

*Cardamom
*Chamomile
*Cinnamon
*Cloves
*Ginger
*Orange Peel

John Douillard's Free Video Newsletter
Your News Source for Ayurveda and Natural Health

Check out the archives of 250+ original articles on natural health and Ayurvedic psychology at LifeSpa.com/articles

Love what you see? You can sign up to receive cutting-edge health updates with an Ayurvedic twist in your inbox every week!
Sign up at LifeSpa.com/newsletter

Services at LifeSpa

John Douillard's LifeSpa
6662 Gunpark Dr E, Suite 102
Boulder, CO 80301
(303) 516 – 4848 or (866) 227 – 9843
lifespa.com | info@lifespa.com

LifeSpa's Mission: To Advance Ancient Wisdom with Modern Science

After studying alternative medicine for the past 30 years with leading experts from around the world, it became clear to me that, while the body is infinitely complex, the best medicine is incredibly simple.

It is my mission to help us transition from a culture of expensive and complex health care to a culture that seeks optimal health through natural mind-body medicine, leaving us more self-sufficient, rather than dependant on a medical system or a pill. ~ *John Douillard*

Ayurvedic Consultations with John Douillard, DC

lifespa.com/consults

John Douillard is available for private consultations in person or over the phone. Through a comprehensive exam aimed at uncovering the cause of what ails you, John Douillard diagnoses and treats the fundamental imbalance that may be responsible for all of your symptoms. Therapies may include, but are not limited to: herbs, diet, exercise, lifestyle changes, and stress prevention.

Panchakarma Rejuvenative Detox Retreats

lifespa.com/panchakarma

Panchakarma is a series of detoxifying, balancing, and nourishing therapies performed over a series of 3, 5, 7 or more days. Panchakarma is not just a detox program. This is only its side benefit. It is a Transformation in consciousness - replacing stress with silence. During your Panchakarma you will receive Ayurvedic spa treatments every day with one or two therapists. You will also meet with John Douillard regularly to unravel old emotions, beliefs, habits, and patterns that contribute to the stress which is typically the under-lying cause of most disease. Each day during your free time you will enjoy a customized practice of rejuvenative yoga postures, breathing techniques, meditation and self-inquiry, along with a special cleansing diet and herbal support. We will send you home with a maintenance plan of herbs, yoga routines, dietary recommendations and stress relief techniques all tailored to your unique needs and goals.

Therapeutic Ayurvedic Spa Treatments

For Relaxation and Rejuvenation

If you live in the Boulder/Denver area or are passing through Colorado, enjoy a 1- or 2-hour Ayurvedic Spa treatment with our loving and skilled Panchakarma therapists. We can design the perfect treatment for you based on your goals, such as detox, sinus decongestion, relaxing muscles, or calming the mind. To book your treatment, simply call our office at 303.516.4848 and let us know what your goals are and we will design the perfect treatment for you!

Self Help Herb Store

store.lifespa.com

LifeSpa offers only the highest quality herbs, nutritional supplements and products to support you on your journey towards optimal health. Our interactive website helps you understand which herbs or supplements will be best for you.

Ayurvedic Skin Care

A Revolutionary Preservative-Free and Chemical-Free Product Line

lifespa.com/skincare

Products that are loaded with preservatives and chemicals are perceived as foreign to the body. This perception by the body triggers an automatic rejection of these products and they are not able to penetrate deep into the tissues. Lifespa skin care products contain no preservative or chemicals. Because of this, the body recognizes Lifespa products as nourishment guaranteeing the deepest possible penetration. At LifeSpa we believe that what you put on your body is as important as what you put in your body. The Skin Care Line includes Himalayan Mist Facial Spritzer, Royal Glow Facial Moisturizer, Fountain of Youth Skin Serum, Crystal Clear Cleanser/Toner, Blooming Lotus Mud Mask and Luscious Mango Body Butter.

What is Your Ayurvedic Body Type and Skin Type?

lifespa.com/healthquiz

Take one of our free interactive quizzes to learn how you can stay balanced and healthy with the best foods, herbs and lifestyle practices for your body type.

Speaking Engagements with John Douillard, DC

lifespa.com/presskit

John Douillard is available to lead workshops, seminars, conferences and lectures. Please contact LifeSpa for more information.

Medical Disclaimer

All material provided from LifeSpa for the Colorado Cleanse is provided for informational or educational purposes only. Schedule a private consult with John Douillard, DC or with a physician regarding the applicability of any opinions or recommendations with respect to your symptoms or medical condition. The instructions and advice presented from LifeSpa for the Colorado Cleanse are in no way intended as medical advice or as a substitute for medical counseling. The information should be used in conjunction with the guidance and care of your physician.

Consult your physician before beginning this program as you would any detox, weight loss or weight maintenance program. Your physician should be aware of all medical conditions that you may have as well as the medications and supplements you are taking.

If you are on diuretics or diabetes medication, have liver or gallbladder disease, take any medications or have any other health concerns, please proceed only under a doctor's supervision. As with any plan, the weight loss phases of this nutritional plan should not be used by patients on dialysis or by pregnant or nursing women.

You must be at least 16 years of age or older to do the Colorado Cleanse.

The Colorado Cleanse is a unique two week home program designed to reset the body's natural detox and digestive function while supporting a gentle detoxification of toxic fat cells.

Acknowledgments

I feel extremely blessed to work with a team here at LifeSpa that deeply cares about the work they do and the people they care for.

This revision of the Colorado Cleanse book has been made possible by the writing skills and wisdom of Katya Slivinskaya and the brilliance and numerous talents of Tauna Houghton. I am so grateful to you both.

I want to also thank Jen Freed for being the final set of eyes to copyedit this book and Nathan Richardson for being a part of our brainstorm team for the Colorado Cleanse revision.

The Colorado Cleanse is such a team effort that I must acknowledge Janaki, Erica, Stacy, Brenda and Tony, whose roles in making the Colorado Cleanse possible are so deeply appreciated.